Vegetarian Revenge

Vegetarian Revenge

Better Living Without Chemistry

by Karen Q:Petersen Mann
with Philip E. Mann, B.Sc., M.D.

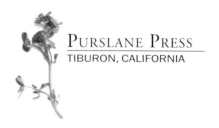

PURSLANE PRESS
TIBURON, CALIFORNIA

Cover Photo:

Tomato Potato Curry, page 167
Spinach Raita, page 26
Banana Raita, page 25
shown served with basmati rice and nan bread

8/2008 Gen Fund 20.⁵

© 2007 Karen Q:Petersen Mann with Philip E. Mann.
Printed in China. All rights reserved.

Although the author and publisher have made every effort to ensure the accuracy and completeness
of information contained in this book, we assume no responsibility for errors, inaccuracies, omissions, or
any inconsistency herein. Any slighting of people, places, or organizations is unintentional.

First printing 2007
ISBN: 978-0-9786295-2-6
LCCN 2006904558

ATTENTION CORPORATIONS, UNIVERSITIES, COLLEGES, AND PROFESSIONAL ORGANIZATIONS:
Quantity discounts are available on bulk purchases of this book for educational, gift purposes, or as premiums
for increasing magazine subscriptions or renewals. Special books or book excerpts can also be created
to fit specific needs. For information, please contact BookMasters, Inc.,
30 Amberwood Parkway, Ashland, OH 44805; (800) 247-6553.

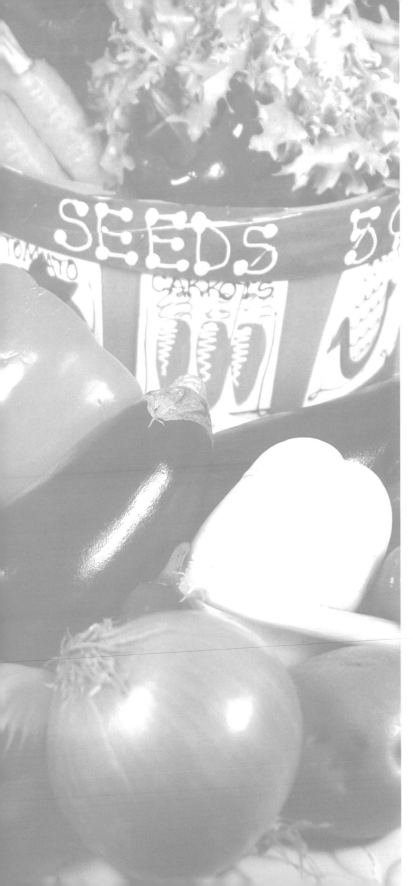

Contents

Introduction

Eating is certainly one of life's principal pleasures. Food preparation—especially when designed to enhance health, prolong life, and increase the quality of life—can be a joyful and fascinating pursuit. Vegetarians outlive flesh-eaters and—by incorporating fruits, vegetables, grains, legumes, and some nuts in their diets—enjoy the beneficial effects of the tocopherols, ascorbic acid, folic acid, and dietary fiber in their food, all of which reduce the risk of cancer, diabetes, and a host of degenerative diseases. A very low-fat diet can be used to correct or ameliorate high cholesterol levels before risking the side effects that can accompany the use of those medications so widely prescribed for that purpose. If a low-fat, reduced-calorie diet is followed, the many ills that obesity brings about are also avoided. That is vegetarian revenge—the revenge of a longer, more robust, and productive existence!

The recipes in this collection are designed to provide low-calorie and very low-fat meals. They compensate for the absence of the flavor-binding and modifying qualities of fat by the use of fresh, organic, unprocessed ingredients, including garlic and other fresh herbs and spices—especially the spices traditionally used in Indian, Mexican, and Far Eastern cooking. The result is flavorful, satisfying food whose aroma and zest can be enjoyed.

The fat used in these recipes is almost exclusively olive oil, the monounsaturated fat of the traditional Mediterranean diet. Eggs are used in muffins, quick breads, and some of the other dishes for their ability to bind ingredients. To a vegetarian or semi-vegetarian who has adapted, high-fat food tastes oily and greasy. This dramatic drop in fat content requires adapting for most, however. The amount of fat used can be doubled for a few weeks at the outset, which may make the transition to ultra-low-fat much smoother.

The composition of an optimum diet is controversial and is currently the subject of heated debate. Everyone's diet consists of a mixture of carbohydrates, fat, and protein, together with nutritionally important phytochemicals and vitamins, but in what proportion? Nutritional scientists have long advised that carbohydrates should supply the majority of calories, while fat and protein comprise the balance. In the final analysis, the total number of calories consumed—no matter at what intervals, at what time of day, and in what composition—determines weight loss or gain. Fat, especially in the form of saturated oils and partially hydrogenated fat, increases the risk of heart disease and probably cancer. In addition, it is a concentrated source of calories—nine calories per gram, while protein and carbohydrates yield four calories per gram. Carbohydrates have historically comprised the major source of caloric intake and should continue to do so.

The recipes offered in this book can be used in a low-calorie diet plan, supplying over 60 percent of total calories in the form of vegetables and grains (i.e., carbohydrates). The addition of salt, which certainly enhances flavor but should be limited because of the risk of hypertension, is left to the discretion of the cook.

Cooking is an art. The same recipe followed by one person may not turn out the same as that prepared by another. Preparation is circled by variables. Gas heat cooks at a different rate than electric. Utensil sizes and composition affect the process. But most important are the ingredients. The best results come from fresh, seasonal, organic vegetables and grains. Obviously, a ripe, juicy, summer tomato results in an entirely different-tasting and -appearing tomato sauce or baked tomato. Recipes should probably be varied, not only with the season and the source, but with the mood of the cook and his or her guests. Recipes really have no beginning and no end; they are part of a continuum seized at one point in time. They are, therefore, to be regarded as starting points, guidelines for further development. This must especially be true of recipes that aspire to high flavor, for the intensity of flavor must suit the individual palate.

Cooking is glorious fun. If it is low-fat and vegetarian, using ingredients uncontaminated with pesticides and chemicals, it gives a sense of achievement and the supreme joy of eating a colorful, healthful, and satisfying meal.

But who should follow a very low-fat diet? Those of us who suffer from elevated total cholesterol, elevated LDL, and reduced HDL lipoproteins. This type of diet should be essayed first before embarking on the lifelong use of cholesterol-lowering agents like the statins. Who else? Those of us who want to lose excess pounds can do so by limiting total calorie intake by eschewing fat—not chewing it—and relying on carbohydrates as the main source of calories. An extensively varied and all-inclusive vegetarian diet should include dairy products, that is, nonfat or low-fat milk, yogurt, and small amounts of cheese and nuts.

Technically, tiny amounts of fat in cooking absolutely require the use of top-quality, nonstick cookware. A mister or spray bottle can be used to distribute oil over the cooking surface. Heating the oil helps to distribute it more evenly, particularly when food is baked or sautéed. If you must, canned, pressurized olive oil may be used.

Fats require more time and effort to digest, so reducing them makes a noticeable difference in the way the eater feels. A low-calorie, low-fat diet may add years to life. Enjoy it!

Diet is of pivotal importance in disease prevention and health, but it must form a part of an overall health-promoting lifestyle. Regular and consistent exercise appropriate to the age and general condition of a person is essential. In addition, stress management, which is dramatically aided by exercise, together with an appropriate diet, completes the plan. A vegetarian diet enhances the enjoyment of eating by freeing one from participation in the abusive, inhumane, and environmentally and personally dangerous practice of reducing living, sensitive animals to the status of a product.

A Few Words About Measurements and Ingredients

Regarding the measurement of recipe ingredients, I have used weights whenever appropriate. Why? Remember standing before the bin of, say, spinach (or green beans or onions) and trying to decide how many bunches of spinach, when chopped, will yield 2 cups? Or how many carrots, sliced or chopped, are right for the recipe you have in mind? Weights, though, like any other measurement method, are rough guides. Use amounts that seem and taste right to you.

Beans are a fine source of protein and fiber, and they are a common ingredient in many of the following recipes. Dried beans have been used in many recipes. Canned—or better, glass-enclosed—beans have been used too. They certainly make a recipe easier and faster to prepare. When you use dried beans, don't use those left over from last year. Stale beans taste pretty good, but they never get tender, no matter how long they cook. Don't waste the time and effort involved in preparing a delicious bean soup, only to find that the beans don't seem to get tender!

Salads

Salads, more than any other food arrangement, must be composed of the very freshest seasonal ingredients. Too long a sojourn in the refrigerator can impair the taste of otherwise superb ingredients.

When using fruit, keep in mind that oranges, grapefruit, and other citrus should be available throughout the year and in high taste. Apples, though, are freshest in fall and early winter: September through November. By August, apples have been in cold storage for eight to ten months, and they taste old. Many varieties are available from the thousands published in botanical journals. Good ones are Gala, Fuji, Cameo, Braeburn, Pink Lady, and Honeycrisp. They vary in crispness and acidity, so suit them to your taste and to the individual salad. For grapefruit, Texas ruby red fruit are often the best and are freshest between December and June. Colorful fruit look best in a fruit salad, and dark red, sweet grapefruit and deep crimson blood oranges leap out.

Fruit Salads

The choice of apples in these fruit salads should suit the cook's taste, but they should be crisp. The apples specified for each salad are suggestions.

Apple-Celery Salad

The brandy and horseradish, though unrelated, marry well in this salad.

¾ cup plain, nonfat yogurt
1 tablespoon cognac or brandy
2 teaspoons horseradish
1 pound Fuji or Pink Lady apples
lemon juice
1 cup celery, chopped

- Whisk together the yogurt, cognac, and horseradish.
- Peel the apples and cut into small pieces. Squeeze some lemon juice over the cut surfaces and combine with the celery.
- Pour the dressing over the apples and celery and stir to combine.

4 servings

Apple-Date Salad

Ripe Medjool dates tend to stick together, so the chopped bits coalesce into a lump. Try separating them after the yogurt is added.

3½ cups Granny Smith apples, cored and cut into ½-inch pieces
lemon juice
5 ounces Medjool dates, pitted and chopped
½ cup celery, chopped
zest of 1 lemon
¾ cup plain, nonfat yogurt
2 teaspoons lemon juice

- Squeeze just enough lemon juice over the apples to coat the cut surfaces.
- Add the dates, celery, and lemon zest to the apples.
- Whisk together the yogurt and the 2 teaspoons lemon juice. Pour over the salad and combine.

4 servings

Apple-Grape-Celery Salad

Choose crisp apples that aren't sour, such as Granny Smith, Fuji, or Pink Lady. You may want to cut the grapes in half to make them easier to eat.

2 cups Granny Smith apples, cored and cubed

lemon juice

2 cups red or green seedless grapes

½ cup celery, chopped

zest of 1 lemon

½ cup plain, nonfat yogurt

2 tablespoons frozen apple juice concentrate, thawed

¼ teaspoon celery seed

- Squeeze a little lemon juice over the apples to coat the cut surfaces.
- Combine the apples, grapes, celery, and lemon zest.
- Whisk together the yogurt, apple juice, and celery seed. Pour over the salad and stir to combine.

4 to 6 servings

Apple-Yogurt Salad

Surprisingly, the taste of the yogurt used in fruit salads is important, since yogurts vary widely in their acidity, fluidity, and flavor. Flavor and consistency should suit your taste. Russian-style yogurts (such as Pavel's) have an almost icy taste and are not uniformly smooth.

½ cup plain, nonfat yogurt

2 tablespoons honey

¼ teaspoon cinnamon

1 pound Granny Smith apples, cored and cut into 1-inch cubes

lemon juice

- Whisk together the yogurt, honey, and cinnamon.
- Squeeze enough lemon juice over the apples to coat the cut surfaces.
- Pour the yogurt dressing over the apples and combine.

4 to 6 servings

13

Apple-Zucchini Salad

Use slender zucchini if you can. Zucchini flavor doesn't improve with aging.

2 Granny Smith apples, peeled and cut into ½-inch cubes

2 cups zucchini, grated coarse

⅓ cup scallions, sliced

¼ cup plus 2 tablespoons plain, nonfat yogurt

2 teaspoons lemon juice

1 teaspoon sugar

1½ teaspoons mayonnaise

pepper

zest of 1 orange

- Combine the apples, zucchini, and scallions.
- Whisk together the yogurt, lemon juice, sugar, mayonnaise, and pepper. Stir in the orange zest.
- Pour over the salad and combine.

4 servings

Orange-Grapefruit-Apple Salad

Elementary indeed, but very refreshing when served with a spicy burger or filet of tofu.

2 ruby red grapefruits
3 large oranges
1 Granny Smith apple
honey

- Juicy, red grapefruit can be peeled by cutting the skin over both poles so the depth of the skin is visible. Cut the skin away from the remaining fruit in a spiral, starting at one pole so the skin and white pith are removed. Do this over a dish to save the juice. Next, cut the fruit into segments between the separating septa.
- Repeat the procedure with the oranges.
- Core and slice the apple thin. Add to the grapefruit and orange sections.
- Add honey, if necessary.

4 servings

Orange-Banana-Grapefruit Salad

The flavor of this salad will vary with the honey used. Try different honeys, such as orange, lavender, millefiori. If the salad is too sweet, vary the amount of lime juice. (See method for sectioning grapefruit in the recipe above.)

4 navel oranges, peeled and sectioned
2 ruby red grapefruits, peeled and sectioned
1 banana, sliced
1 tablespoon honey
1 tablespoon grapefruit juice
1 tablespoon lime juice
3 teaspoons fresh mint, minced

- Combine the oranges, grapefruits, and banana slices in a bowl.
- Combine the honey, grapefruit juice, and lime juice. Pour over the salad and combine.
- Stir in the mint leaves.

4 servings

15

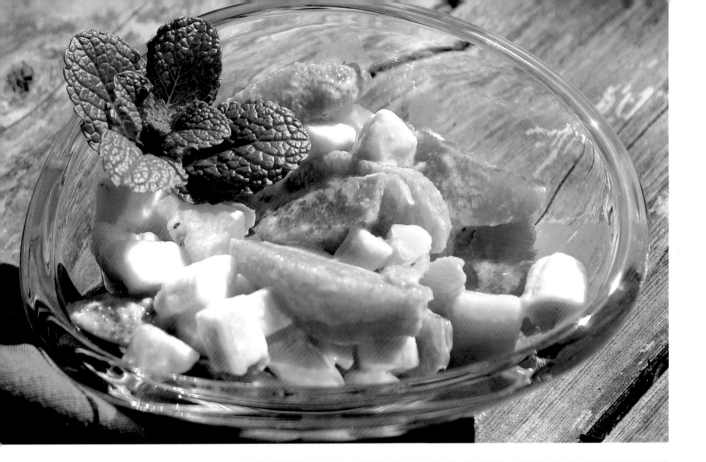

Orange-Kiwi-Banana Salad

Kiwifruit (Chinese gooseberry) is sweet-sour and can taste like strawberries. Its distinctive luminous green color is accented with a circle of dark seeds.

2 kiwifruit, peeled and cut into small cubes

2 navel oranges, peeled and sectioned

2 bananas, peeled and cut into small cubes

¼ cup plain, nonfat yogurt

1 tablespoon lime juice

1 tablespoon orange juice

honey

pinch of nutmeg

- Combine the kiwifruit, oranges, and bananas.
- Whisk together the yogurt, lime juice, and orange juice. Add honey and a pinch of nutmeg. Pour over the fruit and stir to combine.
- Serve immediately.

4 servings

16

Orange-Carrot Salad

Despite the carrots, the flavor of this salad is decidedly fruity. Juicy Valencia oranges, especially if they are tart, dominate the overall flavor. The carrots should be grated with a hand grater to produce small chunks of carrot about ½ inch in length—a bit of crunch to countermand the softness of the orange sections.

2 cups carrots, peeled and grated

1½ cups fresh orange sections, including all the juice

4 ounces red onion, halved lengthwise, sliced, and separated into half rings

½ cup currants, soaked for 30 minutes in dark rum to cover, and drained

⅛ teaspoon crushed red pepper flakes

juice of ½ lemon

pepper

- Combine all of the ingredients and refrigerate 30 minutes or longer before serving.

4 servings

Orange Slices With Cranberry Sauce

The tart-sweet flavor of cranberries, even in summer, makes this a salad worth trying—and a good way to use the frozen cranberries you bought in December.

1 cup sugar

1 cup water

12 ounces cranberries

2 tablespoons Grand Marnier

zest of 1 orange

1 orange per person

mint leaves

- Combine the sugar and water in a pan and bring to a boil, stirring to dissolve the sugar.
- Add the cranberries and cook, partially covered, for 10 minutes, stirring occasionally. Remove from heat and stir in the Grand Marnier and orange zest.
- Cool the sauce.
- Peel the oranges and slice them crosswise. Arrange the slices on individual plates.
- Spoon a small amount of cranberry sauce on top of each sliced orange.
- Garnish with mint leaves.

Serve the remaining cranberry sauce as a condiment with sautéed tofu or marinated tempeh.

Orange-Daikon Salad

Daikon is a member of the radish alliance, usually long and white and rather sweet and juicy. Daikon also usually lacks the sharp bite of red radishes. They are beloved by Asians, but they make a good, crisp salad with Hispanic overtones.

¼ cup lime juice

1 teaspoon chili powder

⅛ teaspoon cayenne

⅛ teaspoon salt

4 navel oranges, peeled and sectioned

4 ounces daikon, peeled and cut into ¼-inch sticks

2 ounces red onion, minced

- Combine the lime juice, chili powder, cayenne, and salt. Let the flavors blend for 30 minutes.
- Arrange the orange sections and daikon on 4 individual plates.
- Sprinkle with the onion.
- Spoon the dressing sparingly over the salads.

4 servings

Cantaloupe Salad

Don't make this salad ahead of time, as it will turn watery. The yogurt dressing should cling to and uniformly coat the chunks of cantaloupe.

1 ripe cantaloupe

¼ cup plain, nonfat yogurt

1 tablespoon honey

1 tablespoon lime juice

¼ teaspoon ground cardamom

- Cut the cantaloupe in half and remove the seeds. Peel and cut the melon into 1-inch cubes. Drain in the refrigerator for 20 minutes.
- Whisk together the remaining ingredients and mix with the melon just before serving.

4 servings

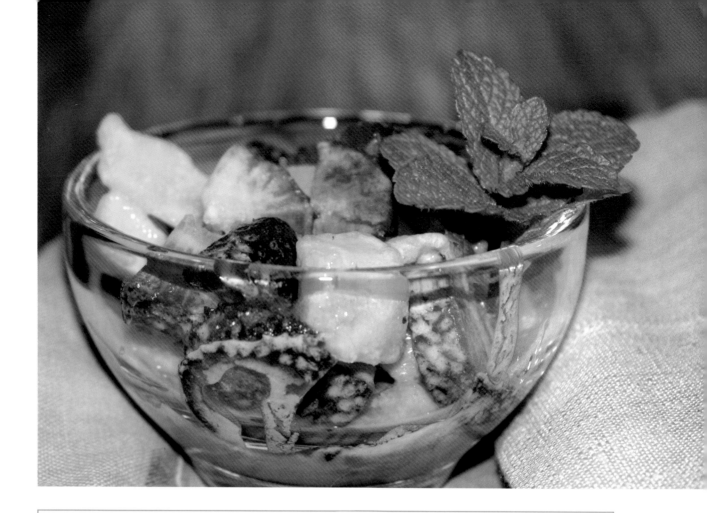

Strawberry-Cantaloupe Salad

This is a sweet salad, but it tastes wonderful with a vegetarian polenta dish.

½ cantaloupe, seeded, peeled, and cut into 1-inch cubes

1½ cups strawberries, sliced

¼ cup plain, nonfat yogurt

1 tablespoon lime juice

1 tablespoon honey

¼ teaspoon cardamom

mint leaves

- Combine the cantaloupe and strawberries.
- Whisk together the yogurt, lime juice, honey, and cardamom. Pour over the salad and stir to combine.
- Garnish with a few mint leaves.

4 servings

19

Grapefruit-Endive-Pomegranate Salad

Belgian endive, the leafy top that can be grown on the humble chicory root, has a rather subtle, bitter flavor that is often obscured by the acidity of lemon juice. Here, the mild acidity and sweetness of the ripe, juicy grapefruit enhance that flavor. The crunchiness of the pomegranate seeds, together with their rich crimson color, adds to the panache of the dish.

2 ruby red grapefruits, peeled and sectioned, seeds removed and the juice reserved

3 endives, sliced crosswise ¼ inch thick

¾ cup pomegranate seeds

1 teaspoon olive oil

½ cup plus 2 tablespoons grapefruit juice

2 tablespoons cider vinegar

2 teaspoons Dijon mustard

pepper

- Holding the grapefruit over a bowl to catch the juice, peel and cut into sections. Add the sections to the juice, using the same technique as in the orange-grapefruit-apple salad on page 15.
- Mound the endives in the center of each of 4 plates. Arrange the grapefruit sections around the endive in spiral fashion. Top with the pomegranate seeds.
- Whisk together the olive oil, grapefruit juice, vinegar, Dijon mustard, and pepper.
- Divide the dressing evenly among the salads.

4 servings

Peach-Celery Salad

Don't use very ripe peaches; they should be ripe and juicy but not mushy so they retain their peachy integrity. The celery should be chopped or sliced so the salad will contrast its crunch with the luscious texture of the ripe peach.

3 large peaches (1½ pounds), peeled and sliced

½ cup celery, chopped

¼ cup plain, nonfat yogurt

1 tablespoon lime juice

1½ teaspoons honey

⅛ teaspoon cinnamon

- Combine the peaches and celery.
- Whisk together the yogurt, lime juice, honey, and cinnamon.
- Pour the dressing over the salad and combine.

4 servings

Pear-Celery-Pomegranate Salad

Pomegranates are fascinating. Their hard, robust exterior conceals lacunae of fleshy, bright red seeds. Try removing the seeds under water in a large bowl to avoid staining your clothing. Drain the seeds in a sieve. The celery and pomegranate seeds add crunch, while the pear should be a bit firm but lusciously yielding.

2 ripe pears, peeled, cored, and cut into large pieces

1 large celery stalk, chopped

½ cup pomegranate seeds

¼ cup plain, nonfat yogurt

1 tablespoon lime juice

1 tablespoon honey

¼ teaspoon cardamom

- Combine the pears, celery, and pomegranate seeds in a bowl.
- Whisk together the yogurt, lime juice, honey, and cardamom. Pour over the salad and mix gently to combine.

4 servings

Pear-Grapefruit Salad

The very best, juiciest, and sweetest grapefruit come from Texas. Frank Lewis, among others, is a good source. Keep the pears immersed in the grapefruit juice until you are ready to serve this dish, to prevent browning. (See method for sectioning grapefruit on page 15.)

Salad:

2 ruby red grapefruit, peeled and sectioned, juice reserved

2 pears, peeled, sliced, and dipped into the grapefruit juice

Dressing:

5 tablespoons grapefruit juice

¼ teaspoon olive oil

1 tablespoon cider vinegar

1 teaspoon Dijon mustard

pepper

cilantro, chopped, for garnish

- Arrange the grapefruit sections and pear slices equally on 4 salad plates.
- Whisk together the dressing ingredients and pour over the salads.
- Add pepper and garnish with the cilantro.

4 servings

21

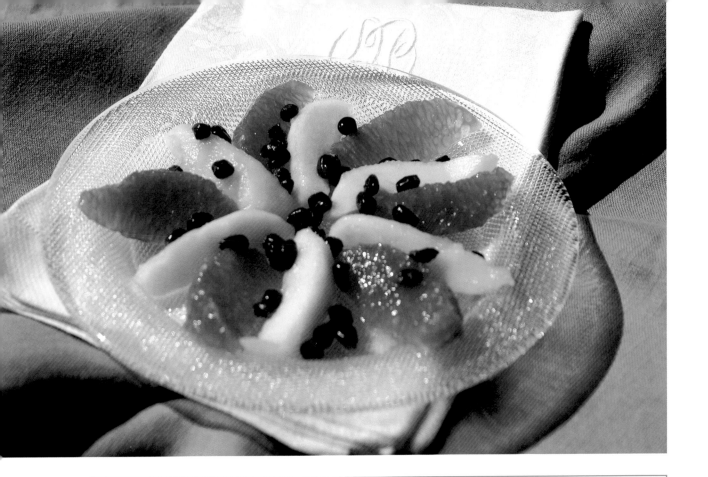

Pear-Grapefruit-Pomegranate Salad

Pomegranates are available in the fall, roughly from September to December. They add brilliant color and a piquant flavor to citrus. (See method for sectioning grapefruit on page 15.)

2 ruby red grapefruits, peeled, sectioned, and seeded, juice reserved

2 ripe pears, peeled, cored, cut into small wedges, and dipped into grapefruit juice

1 cup pomegranate seeds

7 tablespoons grapefruit juice

1 tablespoon cider vinegar

1 teaspoon Dijon mustard

pepper

- Arrange the grapefruit sections and pear slices alternately in spiral fashion on 4 salad plates. Top each salad with ¼ of the pomegranate seeds.

- Whisk together the grapefruit juice, vinegar, and Dijon. Pour equal amounts over the 4 salads. Add pepper.

4 servings

Mixed Summer Fruit Salad (Pico de Gallo)

The simplicity of this fruit mixture preserves and emphasizes the flavor of fresh, full-flavored midsummer fruit. Use appropriate amounts of some or all of the following fruits and vegetables:

honeydew melon, seeded, peeled, and sliced

cantaloupe, seeded, peeled, and sliced

watermelon, seeded, peeled, and cut into wedges

papaya, seeded, peeled, and sliced

cucumber, peeled, and sliced

lime wedges to squeeze over the fruit

chili powder

salt

- Arrange a desired combination of chilled fruit and vegetables on individual serving plates along with lime wedges.
- Along with each serving, provide chili powder and salt, not mixed, for dipping.

Fruit Salad—Looped

Wow! What a salad! The fragrance of juniper berries in the gin ally with the triple sec to produce a unique flavor. Eat this carefully, though; it is potent!

2 tablespoons honey

¼ cup lime juice

5 cups assorted fruit such as berries, peaches, oranges, grapefruit, apples, bananas, nectarines, grapes, and cantaloupe, cut into bite-size pieces

⅓ cup triple sec

⅓ cup gin

2 tablespoons fresh mint leaves, chopped

- Combine the honey and lime juice in a small pan. Bring to a simmer, stirring. Remove from heat and cool.
- Prepare the fruit and place it in a large bowl. Include any juice from the fruit.
- Add the honey and lime mixture along with the triple sec and gin.
- Combine and refrigerate for 45 minutes.
- Stir in the mint leaves just before serving.

4 to 6 servings

23

Fruit Salad With Raspberry Dressing

This is a much more mild-mannered salad. The rum should be dark Jamaican, which merely adds to and modifies the flavor of the sugar.

1¼ cups fresh raspberries
2 tablespoons rum
1 to 3 tablespoons granulated sugar
1 cup fresh blueberries
2 bananas, sliced
1 tablespoon fresh mint, chopped

- Purée ¾ cup raspberries, rum, and sugar.
- Combine the remaining ½ cup raspberries, blueberries, bananas, and mint.
- Pour the dressing over the fruit and stir gently to combine.

4 servings

Fruit Salad With Curried Yogurt Dressing

Here the quality of the curry powder is of crucial importance. Commercially prepared curry powders vary greatly in "heat" and spice content. Choose an Indian powder if you can.

2 nectarines, peeled and cut into pieces
1 cup blueberries
1 cup strawberries, sliced
1⅓ cups red or green seedless grapes, halved
½ cup plain, nonfat yogurt
½ teaspoon curry powder
1 tablespoon lime juice

- Combine the nectarines, blueberries, strawberries, and grapes.
- Whisk together the yogurt, curry powder, and lime juice. Combine with the fruit.

6 servings

Indian Banana Salad (Banana Raita)

Raitas are Indian yogurt salads. This one is cool and refreshing and can be used as a dessert or even with curry as a cooling condiment. This particular Indian "salad" profits from the use of cardamom, a distinctly flavored, aromatic Indian spice. The bananas should be firm-ripe.

1 cup plain, nonfat yogurt
1 tablespoon honey
1 tablespoon lime juice
$\frac{1}{8}$ teaspoon ground cardamom
$\frac{1}{4}$ cup dates, chopped
2 cups bananas, cut into small pieces

- Whisk together the yogurt, honey, lime juice, and cardamom.
- Stir into the dates and chill for 30 minutes.
- Mix in the bananas just before serving.

3 to 4 servings

Grape Salad

With crisp, seedless red grapes, this elementary salad can be refreshing indeed, especially with a tangy, not too sweet yogurt.

$2\frac{1}{2}$ cups red seedless grapes, halved
1 cup plain, nonfat yogurt, whisked
    until smooth
zest of 1 orange

- Combine the grapes, yogurt, and orange zest.

5 servings

25

Vegetable Salads

Spinach Raita

This is another Indian yogurt salad. Increase its impact, if you like, by adjusting the cayenne pepper, or better yet, by using all or part of a small, dried red chili. Toasting the coriander and cumin seeds enhances their flavors and especially their wonderful aromas. Chop the spinach into small bits to make the salad more appealing and easier to eat. This salad is a good match for Tomato-Potato Curry (page 167).

8 ounces spinach leaves, chopped

¾ cup plain, nonfat yogurt

½ teaspoon coriander seeds, toasted and ground

¼ teaspoon cumin seeds, toasted and ground

$1/16$ teaspoon cayenne

salt

- Cook the spinach, covered, over medium-low heat until tender (4 to 6 minutes).
- Drain the spinach and squeeze out the excess water. Cool.
- Whisk together the yogurt, coriander, cumin, and cayenne. Stir in the spinach.
- Add salt.

4 servings

Artichoke Citrus Salad

Choose a juicy, sweet orange that is in season. It may be a navel, a Valencia, or even a blood orange.

½ teaspoon olive oil

5 large garlic cloves, minced

8 fresh, large artichoke hearts, cooked and cut into eighths (see Artichoke Hearts Sautéed With Wine on page 100)

2 lemons: Zest 1, peel it, and cut it into rounds; quarter the rounds and remove the seeds. Juice the other lemon.

3 navel oranges: Zest 1 and juice it. Peel the remaining 2 oranges and cut them into rounds; quarter the rounds and remove the seeds.

¹/₁₆ teaspoon cayenne

pepper

- Heat the olive oil over low heat, add the garlic, and sauté for 1 minute.
- Add the artichokes, citrus, cayenne, and pepper.
- Cook gently for 5 minutes.
- Serve warm or at room temperature.
- For the best flavor, make a day ahead.

4 servings

Asparagus With Citrus Dressing

Choose tender, spring asparagus, preferably from California's new crop (March through early June).

1 pound asparagus, tough ends snapped off, lower stems peeled

¼ cup orange juice

3 tablespoons lime juice

2 teaspoons shallots, minced

1 teaspoon olive oil

1 tablespoon white wine vinegar

2 tablespoons orange zest

- Steam the asparagus until crisp-tender, 3 to 5 minutes. Chill.
- Whisk together the orange juice, lime juice, shallots, olive oil, and vinegar.
- Divide the asparagus evenly among 4 plates. Pour some of the dressing over each serving.
- Sprinkle the orange zest over the salads.

4 servings

27

Asparagus and Tomato Salad

The eternal question: to peel or not to peel. It depends partly on one's taste and partly on the toughness of the asparagus stalk. You can usually detect tough asparagus when you break off the lower stalks. Avoid stalks that are yellow or woody.

1 pound trimmed asparagus
2 tomatoes, cut into wedges
2 tablespoons balsamic vinegar
¼ cup water
1 teaspoon olive oil
2 tablespoons lime juice
4 teaspoons Dijon mustard
1 teaspoon garlic, minced
pepper

- Steam the asparagus until crisp-tender, 3 to 5 minutes. Chill.
- Arrange the asparagus and tomatoes on 4 plates.
- Whisk together the vinegar, water, olive oil, lime juice, mustard, and garlic. Spoon the desired amount of dressing over the salads.
- Add pepper.

4 servings

Asparagus and Tomato Salad With Mexican Dressing

Citrus dressings seem to give low-fat salads good flavor in spite of the absence of oil.

1½ pounds trimmed asparagus
1 cup plain, nonfat yogurt
2 tablespoons fresh orange juice
3 tablespoons fresh lime juice
⅛ teaspoon ground cumin
1 small garlic clove, minced
3 tablespoons cilantro, chopped fine
jalapeño, minced
3 tomatoes, each cut into 6 to 8 wedges

- Steam the asparagus until crisp-tender, 3 to 5 minutes. Chill.
- Whisk together the yogurt, orange juice, lime juice, and cumin. Stir in the garlic, cilantro, and jalapeño.
- Arrange the asparagus and tomatoes on 6 individual salad plates.
- Spoon the dressing over the salads.

6 servings

Garbanzo Bean Salad

Garbanzo beans are a good source of protein, such that each generous portion can contain two grams of high-quality protein. Spicy Dijon, together with a soupçon of garlic, will make the salad a flavorful companion for a crusty baguette and a glass of Beaujolais Nouveau or Merlot.

2 15-ounce cans low-salt garbanzo beans, chilled, rinsed, and drained

4 ounces red onion, chopped

8 radishes, sliced

½ cup celery, chopped

2 tablespoons parsley, chopped

¾ cup plain, nonfat yogurt

2 teaspoons Dijon mustard

2 tablespoons lemon juice

1 teaspoon minced garlic

salt

pepper

- Combine the garbanzo beans, onion, radishes, celery, and parsley.
- Whisk together the yogurt, mustard, lemon juice, and garlic.
- Pour the yogurt mixture over the salad and combine.
- Add salt and pepper.

6 to 8 servings

Black Bean Salad

A hearty salad, very easy to prepare, and best made several hours or more in advance. Don't overcook the beans; they should retain a bit of "bite." The added crunch of the red pepper and celery makes the dish seem more like a salad. The dish can be served warm or cold.

8 ounces black beans, sorted and rinsed

8 cups water

1 teaspoon salt

½ cup celery, chopped

½ cup scallions, sliced

1 cup red pepper, chopped

⅓ cup cilantro, chopped

4 tablespoons red wine vinegar

2 tablespoons lemon juice

1 teaspoon olive oil

salt

pepper

- Bring the black beans, water, and salt to a boil. Reduce the heat and simmer, uncovered, for 1 hour or until done. Drain, rinse, and chill.

- Combine the beans, celery, scallions, red pepper, and cilantro.

- Whisk together the vinegar, lemon juice, and olive oil. Pour over the beans and combine.

- Add salt and pepper.

6 to 8 servings

Garbanzo Bean and Roasted Red Pepper Salad

If the available Roma are depressingly lacking in flavor and juice—hard little flattened ovals—use canned tomatoes (Muir Glen is the brand of choice). Save their juice for pasta sauce.

2 pounds red peppers seeded and cut into 1-inch pieces

1 cup Roma tomatoes, peeled and chopped (10 ounces)

4 large garlic cloves, minced

2 15-ounce cans low-sodium garbanzo beans, drained and rinsed

4 ounces red onion, chopped

⅓ cup balsamic vinegar

salt

pepper

¼ cup fresh basil, chopped

- Combine the peppers, tomatoes, and garlic. Spread the mixture evenly onto a lightly oiled baking sheet with a rim.
- Broil until the peppers soften and begin to char, stirring often, about 35 minutes. Cool.
- Combine the garbanzo beans, onion, vinegar, and pepper mixture.
- Refrigerate for 2 to 3 hours, or preferably overnight.
- Add salt and pepper. Stir in the basil.
- Bring to room temperature before serving.

6 servings

Black Bean and Bulgur Salad

This is another very good bean salad, which also should be made in advance of its use. For this salad, freshly squeezed orange juice and orange zest add greatly to the flavor. Red onion can be used and adds to the appearance of the combination.

8 ounces black beans, sorted and rinsed

1 teaspoon salt

1¼ cups boiling water

1 cup bulgur

2 cups cucumbers, peeled, seeded, and chopped

4 ounces mild onion, chopped fine

zest of 1 large orange

½ cup orange juice

1 teaspoon olive oil

2 tablespoons apple cider vinegar

salt

pepper

- Put the black beans and 1 teaspoon salt into a pot and add enough water to cover by several inches. Bring to a boil, reduce the heat, and simmer, uncovered, until done, 1 to 1¼ hours. Add additional water as necessary to keep the beans covered. Drain, rinse, and chill the beans.

- Pour the boiling water over the bulgur, cover, and let sit for 30 minutes. Fluff with a fork and chill.

- Combine the beans, bulgur, cucumber, onion, and orange zest.

- Whisk together the orange juice, olive oil, and vinegar. Pour over the salad and combine.

- Add salt and pepper.

8 servings

Kidney Bean Salad

Kidney beans give this salad an entirely different flavor from black beans—a lighter, almost fruity, quality. If possible, use beans that have been packed in glass jars; it makes for a less metallic taste.

1 16-ounce can low-sodium kidney beans, drained and rinsed

$^1/_3$ cup celery, chopped

3 ounces red onion, chopped

$^1/_3$ cup red pepper, chopped

freshly ground pepper

1 teaspoon fruity olive oil

2 tablespoons red wine vinegar

2 tablespoons rice vinegar

1 garlic clove, minced

$^1/_4$ teaspoon oregano or, better, at least 1 tablespoon fresh oregano, the Greek variety, if possible

2 tablespoons parsley, chopped

- Combine the beans, celery, onion, and pepper.
- Whisk together the olive oil, vinegar, garlic, and oregano. Pour the dressing over the bean mixture and combine. Refrigerate for at least 2 hours, or for best taste, overnight.
- Stir in the parsley just before serving.

3 to 4 servings

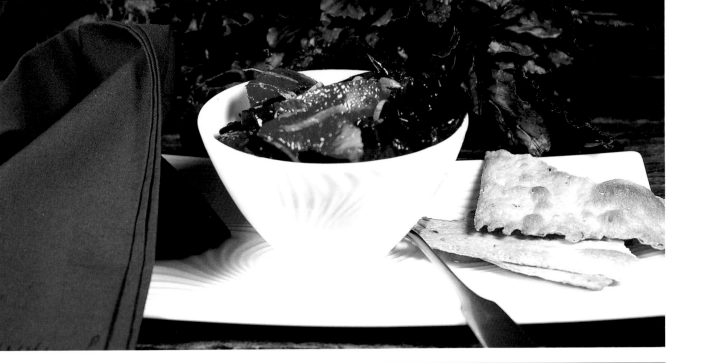

Beet and Orange Salad

Beets make a bloody mess when peeled. Try briefly immersing them in cold water immediately after baking. This may be done in the sink. Beets peel a bit more easily when they are still warm. Choose young beets, if possible, as they are less pungent.

½ pound beets
3 navel oranges, peeled and sectioned
2 ounces red onion, chopped
¼ cup plain, nonfat yogurt
1 tablespoon orange juice
1 teaspoon honey
zest of 1 orange

- Cut off the beet stems, leaving 1 inch. Scrub the beets and bake them, covered, at 375°F until tender, 40 to 45 minutes.
- When cool enough to handle, peel the beets and chill them.
- Coarsely shred the beets with a 6- by 6-millimeter disc in a food processor or by hand. Combine with the oranges and onion.
- Whisk together the yogurt, orange juice, and honey. Pour over the salad and combine.
- Garnish with the orange zest.

4 servings

34

Beet Salad—Pernod

The Pernod adds a characteristic licorice soupçon.

1½ pounds beets, with stems
    trimmed to 1 inch
salt
3 tablespoons balsamic vinegar
4 tablespoons red wine vinegar
1½ teaspoons Pernod

- Scrub the beets and bake them, covered, at 375°F until tender (40 to 45 minutes). Cool, peel, and slice the beets thin. Add salt.
- Mix the vinegar and Pernod with the beets and chill for 3 hours or overnight, stirring occasionally.

4 to 6 servings

Carrot Salad With Black Mustard Seed

Popped black mustard seeds turn gray and give this salad an unusual zest. Put the mustard seeds directly in the small circle of oil before heating so the seeds will be in contact with the oil. Grapeseed oil has a higher smoke point than olive oil, which makes it a better choice for popping the mustard seed.

10 ounces carrots
1 teaspoon grapeseed oil
2 teaspoons black mustard seed
2 teaspoons lemon juice
salt

- Peel the carrots and grate them by hand. Use a medium grater.
- Put the grapeseed oil and the mustard seed in a small covered pan. Heat over medium heat, shaking the pan frequently, until the seeds begin to pop. Reduce the heat and wait until the seeds have all popped (a few minutes). Be careful not to burn them. When the seeds have completely popped, mix them immediately with the carrots.
- Mix the lemon juice with the carrots and add salt.

2 servings

35

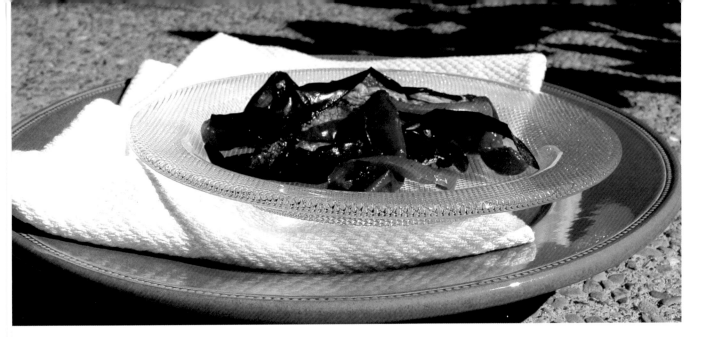

Eggplant-Pepper Salad

Roasting vegetables enriches their flavor, adding a caramel-like taste. Don't roast the vegetables on a sheet pan, as they will burn. Use a heavy cast-iron or ceramic pan.

1 pound eggplant
1 large red pepper
1 large green pepper
6 large garlic cloves, unpeeled
1 teaspoon olive oil
$\frac{1}{3}$ cup red wine vinegar
$\frac{1}{2}$ teaspoon ground cumin
$\frac{1}{8}$ teaspoon cayenne
$\frac{1}{4}$ teaspoon salt
pepper

- Cut the eggplant and peppers into ½-inch strips.
- Combine the eggplant, peppers, garlic, and olive oil in a shallow baking dish.
- Bake, uncovered, at 450°F for 50 minutes, stirring every 10 minutes.
- Remove the garlic and set it aside.
- Transfer the vegetables to a bowl.
- Peel the garlic cloves and combine with the vinegar, cumin, cayenne, salt, and pepper in a food processor. Purée and pour the dressing over the vegetables. Combine.
- Refrigerate overnight.

4 to 6 servings

Green Bean Salad

Use Blue Lake beans that don't look too pregnant. Snap them in half before you buy them. They should be crisp, not rubbery, and should show moisture on the exposed ends.

1 pound green beans, ends removed and broken into 2-inch lengths
4 ounces red onion, chopped
1 large garlic clove, minced
1 tablespoon low-sodium soy sauce
3 tablespoons white wine vinegar
½ teaspoon fresh ginger, grated

- Boil the beans until tender, 5 to 10 minutes. Drain and refresh with cold water.
- Combine the beans with the onion.
- Whisk together the garlic, soy sauce, vinegar, and ginger, and pour over the beans. Stir to combine. Chill.

4 to 6 servings

Green Bean and Cherry Tomato Salad

Eden makes a lower-sodium hot pepper sesame oil. The oil should be the more pungent, toasted oil. This salad can also be served hot, in which case, heat the oil-soy mixture and tomatoes in a pan, gently, and add the still-warm beans. Stir to coat the beans and tomatoes. Heat briefly and serve. Tiny cherry tomatoes work best in this case.

1 pound green beans
1 teaspoon sesame chili oil
½ teaspoon low-sodium soy sauce
1½ cups cherry tomatoes, halved
salt
rice vinegar

- Boil the beans until tender, about 5 to 10 minutes.
- Combine the chili oil and soy.
- Combine green beans, tomatoes, chili oil, soy, and a bit of salt.
- Sprinkle lightly with vinegar.

6 servings

41

Mexican Salad

Corn, tomatoes, jalapeño, and cilantro—especially the cilantro—make this a zingy delight.

corn tortillas, cut into triangles and toasted until crisp; or use purchased fat-free corn chips

2½ pounds tomatoes, cut into small pieces and drained for 15 minutes

3 ounces red onion, chopped

½ cup celery, chopped

1 large garlic clove, minced

½ cup cilantro, chopped

1 ear corn, kernels cut from the cob

jalapeño, chopped

2 tablespoons red wine vinegar

1 teaspoon olive oil

salt

- Preheat oven to 400°F.
- Cut each round of corn tortilla into about 8 sectors. Arrange them on a cookie sheet and crisp in a 400°F oven for about 8 to 10 minutes.
- Combine the tomatoes, onion, celery, garlic, cilantro, corn kernels, and jalapeño.
- Whisk together the vinegar and olive oil. Pour over the salad and stir to combine.
- Add salt and serve immediately with chips.

6 to 8 servings

Fresh Pea Salad

Fresh English peas should be used for this combination. Use small peas that retain some of their mild flavor—those that will cook in a few minutes.

2½ cups fresh peas

½ cup celery, chopped

¼ cup scallions, sliced

½ cup plain, nonfat yogurt

2½ teaspoons Dijon mustard

1½ cups cherry tomatoes, quartered

salt

pepper

- Boil the peas until tender, 3 to 12 minutes. Drain and refresh under cold water. Chill.
- Combine the peas, celery, and scallions.
- Whisk together the yogurt and mustard. Pour over the salad and stir to combine.
- Stir in the cherry tomatoes and add salt and pepper.

6 servings

Potato Salad

Yes, it is possible to make a flavorful, well-lubricated potato salad without slathering it with fat. Here the mayonnaise flavors the yogurt. The acidity, sweetness, and overtones resulting from the species of Lactophilus in the yogurt are important. Tiny red potatoes or waxy-fleshed varieties such as Yukon Gold or Yellow Finn—any of the thin-skinned types—can be used.

2 pounds White Rose potatoes, scrubbed

2 stalks celery, chopped

¼ cup scallions, sliced

1 large carrot, peeled and grated coarse

2 tablespoons parsley, minced

¾ cup plus 1 tablespoon plain, nonfat yogurt

1 tablespoon mayonnaise

1½ teaspoons dry mustard

1 tablespoon apple cider vinegar

5 tablespoons sweet pickles, chopped

salt

pepper

- Cut the potatoes into 1-inch pieces and steam them until tender, about 12 minutes. Salt them while still warm. Cool and chill.
- Combine the potatoes, celery, scallions, carrot, and parsley.
- Whisk together the yogurt, mayonnaise, mustard, and vinegar. Stir in the pickles.
- Pour the dressing over the salad and combine.
- Add salt and pepper.

6 servings

German Potato Salad

This potato salad is hot—that is, in temperature, not spice. This is a zingy, flavorful salad. Notice that it contains no added fat.

1½ pounds red potatoes, scrubbed and cut into 1-inch cubes

¼ cup cider vinegar

6 ounces onion, chopped

1 teaspoon sugar

¾ teaspoon salt

¼ cup water

1 teaspoon sauce and gravy (pulverized) flour

1 tablespoon water

½ cup green pepper, chopped

¼ cup parsley, chopped

pepper

- Steam the potatoes until tender, 10 to 12 minutes. Keep them warm.

- In a small pan, heat the vinegar, onion, sugar, salt, and ¼ cup water to boiling. Reduce the heat and simmer for 5 minutes.

- Stir together the flour and 1 tablespoon water. Add it to the vinegar mixture and cook, stirring constantly, until it thickens slightly.

- In a larger pan, combine the potatoes, dressing, green pepper, and parsley. Heat through gently.

- Add pepper.

6 servings

Potato Salad With Basil and Cherry Tomatoes

Perhaps seven or more cultivars of basil are available in many nurseries. Their use can make this salad taste quite different.

2 pounds red potatoes, scrubbed and cut into 1-inch pieces

1½ cups cherry tomatoes, halved

¼ cup fresh basil, chopped

4 ounces red onion, chopped

¾ cup plus 1 tablespoon plain, nonfat yogurt

1 tablespoon mayonnaise

¾ teaspoon dry mustard

2 tablespoons apple cider vinegar

salt

pepper

- Steam the potatoes until tender, 12 to 14 minutes. Add salt and chill.
- Combine the potatoes, tomatoes, basil, and onion.
- Whisk together the yogurt, mayonnaise, mustard, and vinegar. Pour over the salad and stir to combine.
- Add salt and pepper.

6 to 8 servings

Potato Salad With Beer

Try using a malty brew in this recipe. Birra Moretti (Italian), Bass Pale Ale (U.K.), and Harp Lager (also U.K.) are good choices among many alternatives.

1¾ pounds red potatoes, scrubbed and cut into 1-inch pieces

salt

⅓ cup scallions, sliced

½ cup celery, sliced

2 tablespoons parsley, chopped

¼ cup plain, nonfat yogurt

1 tablespoon mayonnaise

2 tablespoons French's mustard

⅛ teaspoon crushed red pepper flakes

¼ cup cold, pale beer

pepper

- Steam the potatoes until just tender, 10 to 12 minutes. Salt the potatoes, cool, and refrigerate for several hours or until chilled.
- Add the scallions, celery, and parsley to the potatoes and combine.
- Whisk together the yogurt, mayonnaise, mustard, and pepper flakes.
- Stir in the beer slowly and pour over the salad. Stir to combine.
- Add pepper.

6 servings

45

Potato Salad With Green Beans

The flavors of fresh dill and tender young green beans yield a fresh, summery taste.

1½ pounds red potatoes, cut into 1-inch pieces

1 teaspoon olive oil

½ pound green beans, broken into 1-inch pieces

¾ cup plain, nonfat yogurt

2 teaspoons fresh dill, minced

3 tablespoons white wine vinegar

8 ounces red onion, sliced

salt

pepper

- Mix the potatoes with the olive oil. Add salt and pepper in a shallow baking dish. Bake at 425°F for 30 to 35 minutes, stirring often until tender. Chill.

- Boil the beans until tender. Drain and rinse with cold water. Chill.

- Whisk together the yogurt, dill, and vinegar.

- Combine the potatoes, beans, and onion. Mix in the dressing. Add salt and pepper.

4 to 6 servings

Slaw

Make the dressing an hour or more in advance so the curry powder and yogurt can get acquainted. For a bit of additional flavor, immerse the currants, which are usually little nuggets, in bourbon (such as Jack Daniel's) for 45 minutes.

4 cups green cabbage, shredded by hand

½ cup celery, chopped

1 cup Granny Smith or Fuji apples, cored and chopped

1 large carrot, grated

⅓ cup currants, soaked in hot water for 30 minutes and drained well

½ cup plus 1 tablespoon plain, nonfat yogurt

1 tablespoon mayonnaise

1 tablespoon lemon juice

¼ teaspoon ground ginger

½ teaspoon curry powder

- Pull off the outer, usually stained, cabbage leaves. Cut out the core and cut the cabbage in half through its poles. Lay the cabbage, cut side down, on the board and slice the head into thin slivers. Chop the slivers so the pieces can be comfortably held on a fork and do not resemble a load of hay.

- Combine the cabbage, celery, apple, carrot, and currants in a bowl.

- Whisk together the yogurt, mayonnaise, lemon juice, ginger, and curry powder.

- Pour the dressing over the salad and combine.

6 servings

Chinese Cabbage Slaw

This more delicately flavored leafy vegetable is also called Napa cabbage. Shred the cabbage by removing the outer leaves and laying the cluster of leaves flat on the cutting board. Next, slice the leaves into narrow shreds. Chop the shreds again crosswise to provide fork-sized pieces, just as with green, crisp-head cabbage.

5 cups Chinese cabbage, shredded by hand

¼ cup dates, chopped

2 teaspoons sesame seeds, toasted

½ cup plus 2 tablespoons plain, nonfat yogurt

1 tablespoon mayonnaise

1 tablespoon lime juice

¼ teaspoon ground ginger

½ cup pomegranate seeds

- Combine the cabbage, dates, and sesame seeds in a bowl.
- Whisk together the yogurt, mayonnaise, lime juice, and ginger.
- Combine the dressing with the salad.
- Stir in the pomegranate seeds.

6 servings

Red Cabbage Slaw With Peas and Carrots

Hand shredding yields a more uniform texture and less wetness of the cabbage. A food processor is faster, though.

4 cups red cabbage, shredded fine by hand

2 cups fresh peas, cooked and chilled

1 large carrot, peeled and grated

2 tablespoons mild onion, chopped

¼ cup plain, nonfat yogurt

1 tablespoon mayonnaise

2 teaspoons white wine vinegar

2 teaspoons Dijon mustard

salt

pepper

- Combine the cabbage, peas, carrot, and onion in a bowl.
- Whisk together the yogurt, mayonnaise, vinegar, and Dijon mustard. Pour over the salad and stir to combine.
- Add salt and pepper.

6 to 8 servings

48

Spinach-Apple Salad With Honey Mustard Dressing

Apples used in salads should be crisp, so use a red Fuji or a Gala. The red color of the apple makes the salad look even more appealing.

4 ounces spinach leaves washed and torn into bite-size pieces

1 red apple, cored and sliced

2 teaspoons honey

2 tablespoons cider vinegar

1 tablespoon water

1 tablespoon onion, minced

1 tablespoon Dijon mustard

salt

pepper

- Put the spinach and apples into a bowl.
- Whisk together the honey, vinegar, water, onion, and Dijon.
- Add enough dressing to the spinach and apples to coat.
- Transfer the salad to individual plates, adding salt and pepper.

4 servings

Tabouli

This is a delicious Middle Eastern dish often served in Lebanon, Syria, and Israel. The taste of the olive oil is vital to the success of this salad. It must be fruity. A good choice would be the Moroccan olive oil Mustapha's extra virgin oil. Balzana oil from California will add additional flavor because of its buttery but peppery flavor.

1 cup bulgur

1¼ cups boiling water

1 cup fresh parsley, chopped

¼ cup fresh mint, chopped

½ cup scallions, sliced

1½ cups cherry tomatoes, halved

1 cup celery, chopped

1 cup cucumber, peeled, seeded, and chopped

2 teaspoons fruity olive oil

¼ cup fresh lemon juice

2 teaspoons cider vinegar

salt

pepper

- Pour the boiling water over the bulgur and stir. Cover and let stand for 30 minutes. Stir and chill.

- Combine the chilled bulgur with the parsley, mint, scallions, tomatoes, celery, and cucumber.

- Whisk together the olive oil, lemon juice, and vinegar. Pour over the bulgur mixture and stir to combine. Add salt and pepper.

6 servings

Tomato and Lettuce Salad With Tomato Dressing

This salad does have lots of zip but no added fat.

¾ cup peeled, puréed tomato, about 8 ounces

2 teaspoons rice wine vinegar

1 teaspoon Angostura Worcestershire sauce

¼ teaspoon celery seed

¼ teaspoon garlic, minced

salt

pepper

2 cups iceberg lettuce, shredded

½ cup celery, chopped

8 cherry tomatoes, halved

- Combine the puréed tomato, vinegar, Worcestershire sauce, celery seed, garlic, salt, and pepper.
- Combine the lettuce, celery, and dressing. Arrange on 2 plates and top with the cherry tomatoes.

2 servings

Vegetable and Fruit Salad

Butter lettuce is distinctive in flavor and texture. The leaves, held loosely, are delicate, especially if the inner leaves are selected.

½ cup plus 4 tablespoons plain, nonfat yogurt

½ teaspoon light olive oil

½ teaspoon curry powder

¼ teaspoon ground ginger

3 ounces butter lettuce, torn into bite-size pieces

1 cup low-sodium garbanzo beans, rinsed and drained

1 Fuji apple, cored and cut into small pieces. Squeeze a little lemon juice on the cut surfaces.

6 canned artichoke hearts, rinsed and quartered

⅓ cup celery, chopped

3 thin slices of red onion, halved and separated into rings

- Whisk together the yogurt, olive oil, and curry powder.
- In a salad bowl, layer the remaining ingredients in the order listed.
- Just before serving, pour the dressing over the salad and combine.

4 servings

Watercress-Carrot Salad

The sweetness of the carrots amends the mild bitterness of the watercress.

3 ounces watercress, leaves and
    tender stems

1 cup carrots, shredded very coarse

1 teaspoon fruity olive oil

2 tablespoons white wine vinegar

4 tablespoons water

2 teaspoons Dijon mustard

1 teaspoon fresh marjoram, chopped

pepper

- Combine the watercress and carrots.
- Whisk together the remaining ingredients, pour over the salad, and combine.

2 servings

Watercress-Endive-Radish Salad

Endive, which is certainly a mild-mannered vegetable, adds textural variety and a bit of crunch. Discard the blemished outer leaves of the endive and lop off the tough stem end before slicing the endive. This and the other watercress salads can act as an antidote to the rich taste of a tofu or tempeh dish. Rice vinegar, which, of course, is much milder, can be used, but use 2 tablespoons.

4 ounces watercress, coarse stems
    removed

8 radishes, sliced

1 endive, sliced

7 tablespoons fresh grapefruit juice

1 tablespoon cider vinegar

1 teaspoon Dijon mustard

pepper

- Combine the watercress, radishes, and endive in a bowl.
- Whisk together the grapefruit juice, vinegar, and Dijon mustard. Toss with the salad and serve on individual plates.
- Add pepper.

4 servings

Watercress-Cauliflower Salad

Cut the cauliflower into pieces small enough to put into your mouth without cutting them. This will make the marinade more effective.

1 teaspoon olive oil

8 tablespoons white wine vinegar

8 tablespoons water

1½ teaspoons Dijon mustard

¼ teaspoon dried tarragon

1 garlic clove, minced

1 pound cauliflower flowerets

6 radishes, sliced

3 scallions, sliced

2 cups loosely packed watercress leaves, tough stems removed

salt

pepper

- Whisk together the olive oil, vinegar, water, mustard, tarragon, and garlic.
- Combine with the cauliflower and marinate in the refrigerator for at least 2 hours.
- Add the radishes, scallions, and watercress to the marinated cauliflower. Combine.
- Add salt and pepper.

6 servings

Watercress-Grapefruit Salad

My son, who was once executive chef of the Convention Center in Seattle, Washington, appropriated this recipe (without permission, I might add) and incorporated it into the center's menu. It was highly successful.

This salad can be made ahead of its serving time. Use the small, tender leaves of watercress if you prefer a less bitter effect. Try substituting arugula for watercress. With the arugula, use 2 large Valencia oranges instead of grapefruit and replace the grapefruit juice with orange juice—*fresh* orange juice. Use the smallest leaves of arugula. Adjust the amount of vinegar in this salad if necessary; with a very sweet grapefruit, 1½ tablespoons work well.

¾ teaspoon fruity olive oil
(For this salad, Nicolas Alziari oil [from France], Denocciolata [from Italy], or Pope Creek Early Harvest [from California] works well.)

8 tablespoons grapefruit juice

1½ tablespoons cider vinegar

1½ teaspoons Dijon mustard

pepper

4 ounces watercress, tough stems removed

2 ruby red grapefruits, peeled and sectioned, the juice reserved

- Whisk together the olive oil, grapefruit juice, vinegar, Dijon mustard, and pepper.

- Toss the watercress with some of the dressing and arrange it in a mound in the center of each of 4 salad plates.

- Arrange the grapefruit sections in spiral fashion around the watercress, dividing them equally among the 4 salads. (See method for sectioning grapefruit on page 15.)

- Spoon some additional dressing on the salads and add pepper.

4 servings

Watercress-Mushroom Salad

Angostura bitters, together with the brandy and Worcestershire sauce, give this salad an unforgettable flavor, one that complements the slight bitterness of watercress.

5 ounces watercress, leaves and tender stems

½ cup shallots, sliced thin

1 teaspoon olive oil

6 ounces mushrooms, sliced

3 tablespoons lemon juice

1 teaspoon white wine vinegar

¾ teaspoon Angostura bitters

2 teaspoons Worcestershire sauce

4 tablespoons brandy

salt

pepper

- Chill the watercress well.
- Sauté the shallots in the olive oil until soft.
- Add the mushrooms and cook slowly until tender but still moist. Add the lemon juice, vinegar, bitters, Worcestershire sauce, brandy, salt, and pepper. Heat quickly and spoon over the watercress, divided equally among 4 plates.
- Serve immediately.

4 servings

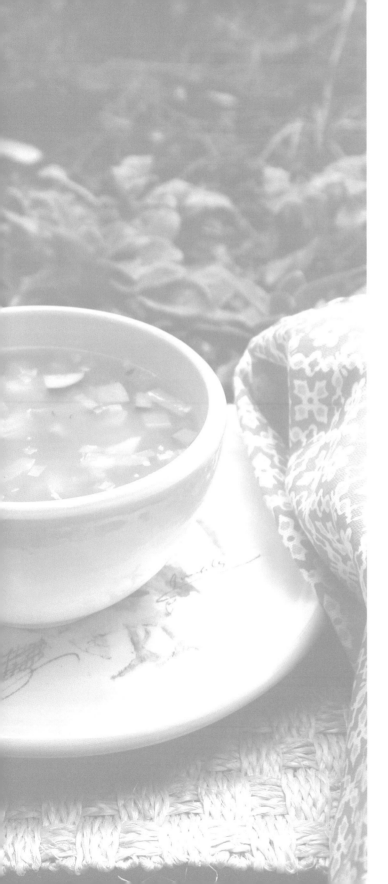

Soups

Food flavors are enhanced by fat and salt. Low-salt cooking, therefore, must be dramatically flavored. The flavors in the following soups, as well as the other vegetarian dishes throughout this book, may seem insipid to you. But remember that flavoring is intensely personal; it is shaped by mood, the time of day, level of fatigue, and the company. Food may taste entirely different, though made according to a recipe, when prepared in a friend's kitchen or when made by another person. The size, shape, and construction of a pan can alter the outcome. Taste the dish, the dressing, the soup, or the pasta before you serve it. Modify the ingredients by adding a bit more oregano or basil or jalapeño. Make the soup or the pasta sauce hours—even many hours—in advance to allow the spices and native vegetable essences to interact and produce an enhanced blend.

A note about broth: Broth is a constituent of many of the recipes in this book—soups and other dishes large and small. Freshly made broth is obviously preferred. Canned and frozen substitutes are available. Swanson makes a canned

(continued)

57

vegetarian broth with a host of best-avoided ingredients: MSG, high-fructose corn syrup, and lots of salt (940 mg in a cup). Healthy Valley, Pacific, and Imagine make organic broth with acceptable ingredients, except for very high sodium levels varying between 350 mg and 530 mg per cup. These are all right if you use only a small volume of the broth, diluted greatly so each serving retains only a small amount of salt. The frozen variety, Rich Vegetable Broth, does not disclose its ingredients.

My son, who is a wonderful chef, tells me that professional chefs sometimes resort to "instant broth"—that is, water. Water can be used in otherwise well-flavored soups and other dishes with acceptable results. Some modification of ingredients may be necessary.

The first broth outlined here is mild, as its headnote states. The second version is more flavorful and can be best used in very mild recipes, such as potato casserole.

Vegetable Broth

This is a rather mild-mannered broth, one that will add to but not overpower the other ingredients.

8 ounces celery, chopped

4 ounces red potato, peeled and chopped

8 ounces peeled carrots, chopped

1 large onion (about 1 pound), chopped

3 large garlic cloves, minced

8 ounces flat-leaf Italian parsley sprigs

1 bay leaf

1½ teaspoons salt

10 cups water

- Combine all the ingredients in a large pot.
- Bring to a boil, reduce heat, cover, and simmer for 1 hour.
- Strain the vegetables from the broth.

7 to 8 cups

A more assertive version of this broth requires the addition of:

¼ cup chopped garlic

3 bay leaves

6 ounces rutabaga, peeled and chopped

6 ounces mushrooms, chopped coarse

2 ounces Hachiya miso

¼ teaspoon red pepper flakes

2 teaspoons garam masala

2 additional cups water

Bean Soup

If you miss the smoky flavor of bacon, the hot smoke flavor of smoked jalapeño chilis or chipotles improves this very easy soup. If you want the soup to sing louder, increase the amount of chipotle or seek out dried peppers in a Mexican market.

2 cups small white beans, sorted and rinsed

8 cups Vegetable Broth (page 58)

¼ teaspoon ground chipotle chili

1½ cups carrots, chopped

½ cup scallions, sliced

1½ pounds tomatoes, washed, stems removed, and chopped coarse

1½ cups water

salt

pepper

chives

3 or more tofu hot dogs, sliced (optional)

- Combine the beans, broth, chipotle chili, carrots, and scallions in a pot. Bring to a boil, reduce heat, and simmer, covered, for 2 hours.

- In a separate pot, cook the tomatoes, covered, for 20 minutes or until soft. Press the tomatoes through a sieve with the back of a spoon to remove the skin and seeds.

- Purée the beans and return them to a clean pot. Stir in the tomatoes and the water. Heat over medium-low heat, stirring frequently.

- Add salt and pepper.

- Garnish with the chopped chives.

- If desired, add the tofu hot dogs and heat before garnishing.

6 servings

59

Black Bean Soup

The more robust flavor of black beans benefits from the more complex flavor of chipotles that have not been imprisoned in a jar.

12 ounces black beans

6 cups Vegetable Broth (page 58)

8 ounces onion, chopped

1 teaspoon olive oil

2 large garlic cloves, minced

1 pound tomatoes, peeled and chopped

¼ teaspoon, at least, dried chipotle chili, cut into small pieces with scissors

1 bay leaf

1 teaspoon ground cumin

½ teaspoon coriander

1 cup red bell pepper, sliced very thin

1 cup celery, cut into small pieces

1 large carrot, grated by hand to yield ¼-inch, flat pieces

salt

pepper

cilantro, chopped

- Bring the beans and broth to a boil, reduce heat, cover, and simmer for 45 minutes.
- Sauté the onion in the olive oil until tender. Add the garlic, briefly stirring.
- Add the tomatoes and cook, covered, until soft (5 to 10 minutes).
- Add the onion and tomato mixture to the beans along with the chipotle, bay leaf, cumin, and coriander. Simmer, covered, for about 35 minutes. Add the red pepper, celery, and carrots to the beans and simmer another 15 minutes or until the beans are very soft.
- Purée 1¾ cups of the soup and return to the pot.
- Heat and add salt and pepper.
- Garnish with the cilantro.

6 servings

60

Many Bean Soup

The variety of beans in this soup gives it a most interesting flavor.

1 large onion (about 1 pound), chopped

3 celery stalks, chopped

1 teaspoon olive oil

4 large garlic cloves, minced

12-ounce variety of dried beans, 1 of each type of bean—pinks, lentils, red kidney, garbanzo, pinto, small whites, Great Northern, black-eyed peas, green split peas, yellow split peas, baby limas, red beans—sorted and rinsed.

8 cups Vegetable Broth (page 58)

1 teaspoon dried thyme

½ teaspoon dried marjoram

½ teaspoon dried rosemary

1 bay leaf

2 pounds tomatoes, peeled and chopped

salt

pepper

parsley, chopped, for garnish

- Sauté the onion and celery in the olive oil until tender. Add the garlic, briefly stirring.

- Add the beans, broth, thyme, marjoram, rosemary, and bay leaf to the pot. Bring to a boil, reduce heat, cover, and simmer until the beans are tender, 1½ to 2 hours.

- Add the tomatoes and cook, uncovered, until the tomatoes are soft (15 to 20 minutes).

- Add salt and pepper.

- Garnish with the chopped parsley.

6 to 8 servings

Chili With Beans and Vegetables

This is a substantial soup, one that can improve if the spices are tweaked with, say, lots of fresh oregano, more cumin, and some of the juicier heirloom tomatoes.

1½ cups pinto beans, sorted and rinsed

1 teaspoon salt

1 pound onion, chopped

1 teaspoon olive oil

4 large garlic cloves, minced

3½ pounds tomatoes, peeled and chopped

½ jalapeño, seeded and chopped

3 tablespoons chili powder

1 tablespoon paprika

1 teaspoon ground cumin

2 teaspoons dried oregano

1 bay leaf

2 cups carrots, chopped

1½ cups green pepper, chopped

2 cups broccoli, chopped

salt

pepper

2 cups zucchini, chopped

- Simmer the pinto beans with the 1 teaspoon salt in enough water to cover by several inches, until tender, 70 to 75 minutes. Add more water as needed to keep the beans covered. Drain and set aside.

- Sauté the onion in the olive oil until tender. Add the garlic, briefly stirring.

- Add the tomatoes, jalapeño, chili powder, paprika, cumin, oregano, and bay leaf to the pot. Cook, covered, until tomatoes are pulpy (about 20 minutes).

- Add the carrots during the last 10 minutes.

- Add the green pepper, broccoli, and beans to the pot. Continue cooking, covered, for 15 minutes.

- Add salt and pepper.

- Add the zucchini and cook 5 minutes.

6 to 8 servings

Chili With Pinto Beans

Despite the relatively strong seasoning in this chili, the tomatoes are the most important ingredient. If they are fresh and juicy, the flavor will be rewarding.

10 ounces pinto beans, sorted and rinsed

1 teaspoon salt

8 ounces onion, chopped

1 teaspoon olive oil

5 large garlic cloves, minced

3½ pounds tomatoes, peeled and chopped

3 tablespoons chili powder

1 teaspoon ground cumin

2 teaspoons dried oregano

1 tablespoon paprika

1½ teaspoons crushed red pepper flakes

1½ cups green pepper, chopped

salt

pepper

1½ cups dry, red wine

cilantro, chopped, for garnish

- Cook the beans and the 1 teaspoon salt in enough water to cover until tender, 65 to 70 minutes. Add more water if necessary to keep the beans covered. Drain and set aside.

- Sauté the onion in the olive oil until beginning to brown. Add the garlic, briefly stirring.

- Add the tomatoes, chili powder, cumin, oregano, paprika, and pepper flakes to the pot. Cook, uncovered, for 15 minutes.

- Add the beans and the green pepper to the pot and continue cooking for 30 minutes.

- Add salt and pepper.

- Stir in the red wine 5 minutes before the dish is done.

- Garnish with cilantro leaves.

6 servings

Minestrone With Beans

Minestrone means "big soup," and this soup is a big, hearty, beany soup containing lots of vegetables—really a full meal in itself.

½ cup small white beans

¼ teaspoon salt

1 large tomato (roughly 1 pound), peeled and chopped

2 large carrots, peeled and chopped

2 large celery stalks, chopped

1 cup cauliflower flowerets

1 teaspoon olive oil

8 cups Vegetable Broth (page 58)

3 tablespoons double-concentrated Italian tomato paste (comes in a tube)

8 ounces red potatoes, scrubbed and cut into 2-inch cubes

4 ounces onion, sliced

¼ head green cabbage, shredded by hand

1 cup fresh peas

½ bunch spinach, chopped fine

2 medium zucchini, chopped fine

salt

pepper

- Cook the white beans with the ¼ teaspoon salt in enough water to cover, until done, 50 to 55 minutes, adding water if necessary. Drain and set aside.

- Sauté the tomato, carrots, celery, and cauliflower in the olive oil for 10 minutes.

- Add the broth, tomato paste, potatoes, sliced onion, cabbage, and peas to the pot. Bring to a boil, reduce heat, cover, and simmer for 10 minutes.

- Add the spinach and zucchini and cook for 15 minutes.

- Add the cooked beans and heat for 10 more minutes.

- Add salt and pepper.

6 to 8 servings

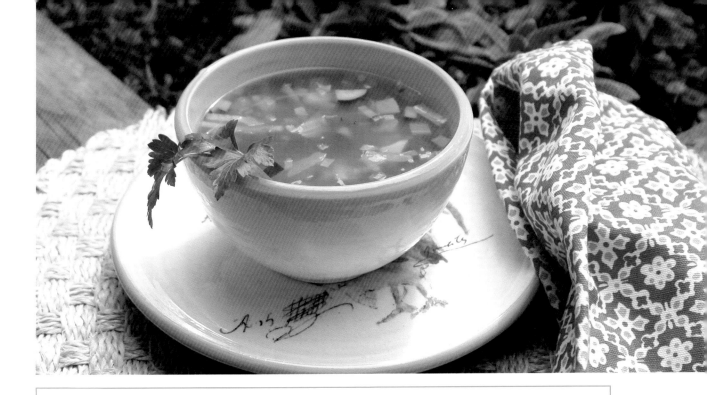

Minestrone With Pasta

The added pasta makes this version substantial.

1 onion (about 8 ounces), chopped

3 garlic cloves, minced

1 cup celery, chopped

1 cup carrots, chopped

1 teaspoon olive oil

8 cups Vegetable Broth (page 58)

4 tomatoes (about 1½ pounds), peeled and chopped

½ teaspoon dried thyme

1½ cups cabbage, shredded by hand

¼ cup spaghetti, broken into 1½-inch pieces

1 cup zucchini, chopped

salt

pepper

- Sauté the onion, garlic, celery, and carrots in the olive oil for 5 minutes.
- Add the broth, tomatoes, thyme, cabbage, and spaghetti to the pot. Bring to a boil, reduce heat, and simmer for 15 minutes or until the spaghetti is just tender.
- Add the zucchini and cook until tender.
- Add salt and pepper.
- Let stand for 6 hours or overnight.

6 servings

67

Lentil Soup

Try using tiny green French lentils, *lentille verte*, available in cans or in bulk in some stores. If you do, you will probably want to use more broth or water to keep the soup at a reasonably good consistency.

1 onion (about 8 ounces), chopped

1 teaspoon olive oil

3 large garlic cloves, minced

3 carrots, peeled and sliced

2 large celery stalks, chopped

12 ounces lentils, sorted and rinsed

8 cups Vegetable Broth (page 58)

$^1/_3$ cup parsley, chopped

½ teaspoon thyme

1 bay leaf

1½ pounds tomatoes, peeled and chopped

salt

pepper

- Sauté the onion in the olive oil until tender.
- Add the garlic, carrots, and celery to the pot and sauté for 5 minutes.
- Add the lentils, broth, parsley, thyme, and bay leaf to the pot. Bring to a boil, reduce heat, and simmer for 1 hour.
- Add the tomatoes and simmer, uncovered, for 20 minutes.
- Add salt and pepper.
- If the soup is too thick, add some additional water.
- The taste improves greatly the second day.

6 to 8 servings

Lentil Vegetable Soup

Cabbage and lentils mate well in this soup. The addition of cabbage makes this a heartier soup.

1 onion, chopped

1 teaspoon olive oil

2 garlic cloves, minced

8 cups Vegetable Broth (page 58)

1 cup lentils, sorted and rinsed

6 ounces peeled carrots, sliced

4 ounces trimmed celery, chopped

2 pounds tomatoes, peeled and chopped

¾ pound red potatoes, scrubbed and cut into 2-inch cubes

½ pound cabbage, shredded by hand

salt

pepper

- Sauté the onion in the olive oil until tender. Add the garlic, briefly stirring.
- Add the broth and lentils to the pot. Bring to a boil, reduce the heat, cover, and simmer for 30 minutes.
- Add the carrots, celery, and tomatoes to the pot. Cook, uncovered, for 25 minutes.
- Add the potatoes and cabbage to the pot. Continue cooking, uncovered, until the vegetables are tender, about 25 minutes.
- Add salt and pepper.

6 to 8 servings

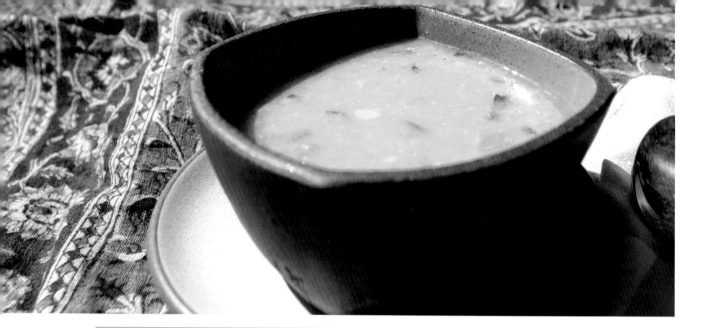

Red Lentil and Carrot Soup

Organic red lentils taste good but do not thicken soup significantly. If you prefer a thick soup, try using less water or buy the lentils from an Indian food source.

8 ounces onion, chopped

1 teaspoon olive oil

3 large garlic cloves, minced

1 teaspoon ground cumin

¼ teaspoon turmeric

1 teaspoon ground coriander

9 cups water

¾ pound red lentils, sorted and rinsed

10 ounces peeled carrots, cut into small pieces

1 cup red pepper, chopped

salt

pepper

cilantro

- Sauté the onion in the olive oil until tender. Add the garlic, briefly stirring.
- Add the cumin, turmeric, and coriander. Stir briefly.
- Add the water and lentils to the pot. Bring to a boil, reduce heat, and simmer, covered, for 70 minutes or until the lentils are done.
- Add the carrots and red pepper and continue cooking, covered, for 5 to 7 minutes or until the carrots are tender.
- Add salt and pepper.
- Stir in the cilantro just before serving.

6 servings

Broccoli Soup

This soup can be delightful or terrible. The broccoli must be young and sweet. Don't use the stems; save them for making broth. A spoonful of tart yogurt gives the soup visual appeal and flavor contrast.

1½ pounds broccoli, chopped

1 pound peeled russet potatoes, chopped

8 ounces onion, chopped

2 teaspoons garlic, minced

6 cups Vegetable Broth (page 58)

1¾ cups nonfat milk

salt

pepper

plain, nonfat yogurt

- Combine the broccoli, potatoes, onion, garlic, and vegetable broth in a pot. Bring to a boil, reduce heat, cover, and simmer for 20 minutes or until the vegetables are tender.
- Purée the soup in several batches until smooth. Return the soup to a clean pot and stir in the milk.
- Heat the soup over medium heat and add salt and pepper.
- Garnish with some plain, nonfat yogurt.

6 servings

Broccoli-Tomato Soup

Fresh, seasonal, organic ingredients are certainly most important in the simpler soups and entrées with only a few ingredients—which are often the best dishes.

12 ounces onion, chopped

1 teaspoon olive oil

1½ pounds tomatoes, peeled and chopped

5½ cups Vegetable Broth (page 58), divided

1 pound broccoli, cut into small pieces

3 tablespoons double-concentrated Italian tomato paste (comes in a tube)

salt

pepper

small basil leaves

- Sauté the onion in the olive oil until soft.
- Add the tomatoes and cook for 5 minutes.
- Add the 3 cups broth and the broccoli to the pot. Bring to a boil, reduce heat, cover, and cook until the broccoli is very tender, about 30 minutes.
- Purée and return to a clean pot. Stir in the tomato paste and the remaining 2½ cups broth. Add additional broth if the soup seems too thick.
- Heat and add salt and pepper.
- Garnish with the basil leaves.

6 servings

Curried Carrot Soup

Select a curry powder that matches your taste for heat and flavor.

2 medium onions (at least 1 pound), chopped

1 teaspoon olive oil

1¼ teaspoons curry powder

1½ pounds carrots, peeled and chopped

2 cups Vegetable Broth (page 58)

4 cups water, divided

½ cup dry sherry

salt

pepper

- Sauté the onion in the olive oil until tender.
- Add the curry powder and cook for 1 minute, stirring.
- Add the carrots, broth, and 1 cup water to the pot. Bring to a boil, reduce heat, and simmer, covered, until the carrots are tender (30 to 40 minutes).
- Purée and return to a clean pot. Add the remaining 3 cups water and the sherry. Heat for 15 minutes, adding salt and pepper.

6 servings

Curried Cauliflower Soup

Curry powder varies greatly in flavor and heat, so choose one that you like, but experiment too.

1 pound onion, chopped

1 teaspoon olive oil

3 garlic cloves, minced

1¼ pounds cauliflower flowerets

1 cup celery, sliced

6½ cups Vegetable Broth (page 58), divided

1½ teaspoons curry powder

salt

pepper

- Sauté the onion in the olive oil until tender. Add the garlic, briefly stirring.
- Add the cauliflower, celery, 4½ cups broth, and curry powder to the pot. Bring to a boil, reduce heat, cover, and simmer for 30 minutes or until the cauliflower and celery are tender.
- Purée and return to a clean pot with the remaining 2 cups vegetable broth.
- Heat, stirring often.
- Add salt and pepper.

6 servings

Curried Crookneck Squash Soup

Small crookneck squash are not as aggressive as some other squash, so this will be a mild-mannered soup to pair with a flavorful salad such as Tabouli (page 50), or Watercress-Mushroom Salad (page 56) or Watercress-Endive-Radish Salad (page 53).

4 large shallots, minced

1 teaspoon olive oil

2 large garlic cloves, minced

2 pounds yellow crookneck squash, cut into 2-inch cubes

3 cups Vegetable Broth (page 58)

¾ teaspoon curry powder

1 cup nonfat milk

salt

plain, nonfat yogurt

chives, chopped

- Sauté the shallots in the olive oil until tender. Add the garlic, briefly stirring.
- Add the squash, broth, and curry powder to the pot. Bring to a boil, reduce heat, and simmer, covered, for 20 minutes or until the squash is tender.
- Purée and return to a clean pot.
- Stir in the milk and heat.
- Add salt.
- Garnish with the yogurt and the chives.

6 servings

Cauliflower-Potato Soup

This, too, is a relatively mild-flavored soup, one that tastes predominantly of cauliflower—a good taste.

1½ pounds cauliflower, cut into 1-inch cubes

12 ounces peeled russet potatoes, cut into 1-inch cubes

8 ounces onion, chopped

6½ cups Vegetable Broth (page 58), divided

⅛ teaspoon cayenne

1¼ teaspoons ground coriander

salt

- In a large pan, combine the cauliflower, potatoes, onion, and 5 cups vegetable broth. Bring to a boil, reduce heat, and simmer, covered, for 20 minutes or until very tender.
- Purée the soup in a food processor and return to a clean pot. Stir in the remaining 1½ cups vegetable broth, cayenne, and coriander.
- Heat through, stirring often.
- Add salt.

6 servings

Corn and Yam Soup

The flavor of yams (sweet potatoes, in the United States), Garnet or Jewel, blends perfectly with the sweetness of summer corn. Avoid corn that has been stored for months and smells and tastes just slightly musky.

1 onion, chopped

1 teaspoon olive oil

3 garlic cloves, minced

2 pounds peeled yams, cut into 1-inch cubes

7½ cups Vegetable Broth (page 58)

1¾ cups fresh corn kernels, steamed for 7 to 8 minutes

salt

pepper

- Sauté the onion in the olive oil until soft. Add the garlic, briefly stirring.
- Add the yams and broth to the pot. Simmer, covered, until tender (about 30 minutes).
- Purée in batches and return to a clean pot.
- Add the cooked corn kernels and simmer, uncovered, for 15 minutes.
- Add salt and pepper.

6 servings

Cold Cucumber Soup

This is a delicious chilled soup, but use firm, homegrown cucumbers if you can. We've used farina (Cream of Wheat cereal) because it thickens easily without forming lumps and tastes better than, say, flour—especially in a cold soup.

1 onion, chopped

1 teaspoon olive oil

2 pounds cucumbers, peeled, halved lengthwise, and sliced

4 cups Vegetable Broth (page 58)

1 tablespoon farina

1 tablespoon fresh dill, chopped fine, or 1 teaspoon dry dill weed

salt

pepper

plain, nonfat yogurt

dill sprigs

- Sauté the onion in the olive oil until soft.
- Add the cucumber and sauté briefly.
- Add the broth, farina, and dill to the pot. Bring to a boil, reduce heat, cover and simmer for 35 minutes or until the cucumber is soft.
- Purée and add salt and pepper.
- Press the soup through a fine sieve to remove cucumber seeds.
- Chill.
- Top each serving with a dollop of yogurt and a dill sprig.

4 to 6 servings

Eggplant Soup

Again, youthful vegetables usually retain more of their character and sweetness, so find small eggplants or some of the slender, torpedo-shaped varieties.

1½ pounds eggplant, sliced thin

1 pound onion, chopped

1 teaspoon olive oil

4 garlic cloves, minced

8 ounces russet potato, peeled and cut into 1-inch cubes

5 cups Vegetable Broth (page 58)

½ teaspoon dried oregano

3 cups water

3 tablespoons double-concentrated Italian tomato paste (comes in a tube)

salt

pepper

cilantro

- Bake the eggplant slices in 1 layer on baking sheets at 375°F for 15 minutes. Cover the baking sheets with foil and continue baking for 30 minutes.
- Sauté the onion in the olive oil until tender. Add the garlic, briefly stirring.
- Add the potato, broth, and oregano to the pot. Bring to a boil, reduce heat, cover, and simmer for 20 minutes or until the potatoes are very soft.
- Purée the potato mixture along with the eggplant slices and return to a clean pot.
- Stir in the water and tomato paste.
- Add salt and pepper.
- Garnish with the cilantro.

6 servings

Gazpacho

A good soup for a hot day! Gazpacho is almost a liquid salad. Serve it with some good whole-grain bread and perhaps a glass of Rioja.

1 generous pound tomatoes, peeled and cut into small pieces

1 cup celery, chopped fine

1 cup cucumber, peeled and cut into small pieces

1 cup green pepper, seeded and cut into small pieces

4 ounces red onion, chopped

¼ cup parsley, minced

3 large garlic cloves, minced

3 tablespoons garlic-flavored red wine vinegar

3 teaspoons Angostura Worcestershire sauce

3 cups tomato juice or V-8–type juice, chilled

cilantro, chopped

- Combine all of the ingredients except the cilantro. Chill for at least 4 hours.
- Serve in chilled bowls and garnish with cilantro.

6 servings

Leek-Broccoli-Spinach Soup

Leeks are full of grit. The onion-like layers of the white parts always seem to conceal sand. So cut the white part in half longitudinally, without separating it from the green part, and then carefully separate the layers while rinsing away the grit. If the soup still is gritty, you will know it was the spinach. Try fresh lemon thyme in place of English thyme, or even Wedgewood thyme if you grow it.

3 cups leeks, pale green and white parts only, washed well and sliced thin

1 teaspoon olive oil

¾ pound broccoli, cut into small pieces

8 ounces russet potatoes, peeled and cut into small pieces

1 tablespoon fresh thyme, chopped

5 cups Vegetable Broth (page 58), divided

2 cups spinach, chopped

½ cup nonfat milk

salt

pepper

chives, chopped

- Sauté the leeks in the olive oil until tender, about 10 minutes.
- Add the broccoli, potato, thyme, and 4 cups broth to the pot. Bring to a boil, reduce heat, cover, and simmer until the vegetables are tender, about 25 minutes.
- Add the spinach and continue cooking, covered, until the spinach is done, about 5 minutes. Purée the soup and return to a clean pot.
- Stir in the remaining 1 cup broth and the milk. Heat the soup, stirring often. Add salt and pepper.
- Garnish with the chives.

6 servings

Mushroom Soup

The mushrooms should be cut into pieces small enough to put into your mouth without cutting them in the soup bowl. Experiment with shiitake or porcini mushrooms. Dried mushrooms can also be used. The flavor of the mushrooms predominates, so try the more flavorful types.

1 onion (about 8 ounces), chopped

1 large celery stalk, chopped

1 teaspoon olive oil

1 pound mushrooms

4 cups Vegetable Broth (page 58)

10 ounces russet potato, peeled and cut into 1-inch cubes

1 cup nonfat milk

3 tablespoons dry sherry

salt

pepper

parsley, chopped, for garnish

- Sauté the onion and celery in the olive oil until tender.
- Add the mushrooms and sauté until almost tender.
- Add the vegetable broth and peeled potatoes to the pot. Bring to a boil, reduce heat, cover, and simmer until the mushrooms are tender, about 30 minutes.
- Add the milk and sherry and heat gently.
- Add salt and pepper.
- Garnish with the chopped parsley.

4 to 6 servings

Mushroom-Barley Soup

In this mushroom soup, the barley flavor coalesces with the mushroom taste, making the resulting flavor much different from the preceding soup.

½ cup barley, rinsed

7½ cups Vegetable Broth (page 58)

8 ounces onion, chopped

1 teaspoon olive oil

2 large garlic cloves, minced

1 pound mushrooms, sliced into bite-sized pieces

4 tablespoons dry sherry

4 tablespoons low-sodium soy sauce

salt

pepper

- Cook the barley slowly in 2½ cups broth, covered, until tender, about 50 to 60 minutes.
- Sauté the onion in the olive oil until tender. Add the garlic, briefly stirring.
- Add the mushrooms and sauté until tender.
- Add the remaining 5 cups broth, barley, sherry, and soy sauce. Bring to a boil, reduce heat, and simmer slowly, uncovered, for 20 minutes. Add salt and pepper.

6 servings

Fresh Pea Soup

Fresh, young peas impart a delicious smoothness that is almost sweet and buttery in flavor.

12 ounces onion, chopped

1 teaspoon olive oil

1 cup celery, chopped

½ cup carrots, chopped

3 cups fresh peas

5 cups Vegetable Broth (page 58), divided

salt

pepper

- Sauté the onion in the olive oil until tender.
- Add the celery, carrots, peas, and 4 cups broth to the pot. Bring to a boil, reduce heat, and simmer, covered, for 15 minutes or until the vegetables are tender.
- Purée and return to a clean pot. Stir in the remaining 1 cup broth.
- Heat and add salt and pepper.

6 servings

Split Pea Soup

Certainly this is one of the simplest soups to put together, and the split peas are rich in flavor because of the close-knit texture of the purée. Passing the soup through the fine disc of a food mill ensures that the texture is smooth and lump-free.

2 cups green split peas

2 large stalks celery, chopped coarse

1 large carrot (about 8 ounces), chopped coarse

1 medium onion (about 6 to 8 ounces), chopped coarse

4 large parsley sprigs

$\frac{1}{8}$ teaspoon cayenne

1 bay leaf

1 teaspoon thyme

8 cups water

2½ teaspoons salt

pepper

- Combine all of the ingredients in a pot and boil for 15 minutes.
- Reduce the heat, cover, and simmer for 1 hour.
- Remove the bay leaf and parsley stems. Put the soup through a food mill.
- Heat over low heat, stirring often. Add some additional water if the soup seems too thick.

8 servings

Split Pea Soup With Sorrel

Sorrel is hard to come by in many markets, but it is a common sight in all 50 states as the curly, yellow, or sour form of the Rumex species: dock. It can be cultivated and in some forms resembles watercress, or in others, has an elongated form. All of the shapes and origins are tart and share the pulsing acidity of spinach, rhubarb, and purslane. The tart flavor adds much to the rather green blandness of split peas. The amount used should be adjusted to your individual taste.

2 cups green split peas, sorted and rinsed

2 stalks celery, chopped coarse

1 large carrot, chopped coarse

1 medium onion (about 6 to 8 ounces), chopped coarse

4 large parsley sprigs

1¾ ounces sorrel leaves, chopped

1 bay leaf

10 cups water

salt

pepper

- Combine the split peas, celery, carrot, onion, parsley, sorrel, bay leaf, and water in a pot. Bring to a boil for 15 minutes.
- Reduce the heat, cover, and simmer for 1 hour or until the peas are very soft.
- Remove the parsley stems and bay leaf and put the soup through a food mill.
- Heat over low heat, stirring often.
- Add salt and pepper.

6 servings

Potato Soup

The potatoes have to be sound, not smelling of mold.

2½ pounds russet potatoes, peeled and cut into 1-inch cubes

8 ounces onion, chopped

6½ cups Vegetable Broth (page 58), divided

salt

pepper

⅓ cup parsley, chopped

- Cook the potatoes, onion, and 5½ cups broth, covered, for 20 minutes or until the potatoes are tender.
- Purée the potatoes and return them to a clean pot along with the remaining 1 cup broth.
- Heat the soup, stirring often, and add salt and pepper.
- Stir in the parsley just before serving.

6 to 8 servings

Vegetable Soup

Again, *fresh*, sweet, and small green beans, the ones that snap off crisply rather than bending obstinately, will make this a truly enjoyable soup.

1 pound onion, chopped

1 cup celery, chopped

1 cup carrots, chopped

1 teaspoon olive oil

4 large garlic cloves

1½ pounds tomatoes, peeled and chopped

11 cups Vegetable Broth (page 58)

¾ teaspoon dried oregano

8 ounces green beans, ends removed and broken into small pieces

12 ounces red potato, scrubbed and cut into small pieces

1 ear corn, kernels cut from the cob

2½ cups cabbage, shredded by hand

1 cup fresh peas

1 cup frozen baby lima beans

3 tablespoons double-concentrated tomato paste (comes in a tube)

salt

pepper

½ cup parsley, chopped

- Sauté the onion, celery, and carrots in the olive oil for 8 minutes. Add the garlic, briefly stirring.

- Add the tomatoes, broth, and oregano to the pot. Bring to a boil, reduce heat, and simmer for 20 minutes.

- Add the green beans and simmer for 15 minutes.

- Add the potatoes, corn, cabbage, peas, lima beans, and tomato paste. Simmer for 15 minutes or until the vegetables are tender.

- Add salt and pepper.

- Stir in the parsley.

8 servings

Vichyssoise

Healthy potatoes are required; make sure they don't smell a bit off (i.e., moldy). A good potato should smell almost sweet when cut. See method for cleaning leeks on page 81.

8 ounces onion, chopped

2 cups leeks, white and pale green parts only, washed well and sliced thin

1 teaspoon olive oil

8 cups Vegetable Broth (page 58)

2 pounds russet potatoes, peeled and chopped

2 cups nonfat milk

salt

pepper

chives, chopped

- Sauté the onion and leeks in the olive oil until tender.
- Add the broth and potatoes to the pot. Bring to a boil, reduce heat, and simmer, covered, until the potatoes are soft, about 20 minutes.
- Purée and cool.
- Add the milk, salt, and pepper. Chill thoroughly.
- Garnish with the chives.

8 to 10 servings

Water Chestnut and Watercress Soup

Some markets carry fresh water chestnuts. Use them if you can. Peel the dark integument from each corm and fine-slice it. Fresh water chestnuts can be used without cooking to add a bit of crunch.

6 cups Vegetable Broth (page 58)

1 tablespoon plus 1 teaspoon low-sodium soy sauce

½ teaspoon sesame oil

1 8-ounce can water chestnuts, rinsed and sliced

2 ounces watercress leaves

- Bring the broth to a boil.
- Add the soy sauce and sesame oil.
- Add the water chestnuts and return to a boil to heat through.
- Add the watercress and simmer for 2 to 3 minutes.

4 to 6 servings

Watercress-Potato Soup

The watercress imparts a soupçon of bitterness and makes the soup sing softly.

1 pound onion, chopped

1 teaspoon olive oil

3½ cups Vegetable Broth (page 58)

2 pounds russet potatoes, peeled and cut into small cubes

2 cups watercress leaves (about 1 large bunch of watercress)

1¾ cup nonfat milk

salt

pepper

watercress sprigs for garnish

- Sauté the onion in the olive oil until tender.
- Add the broth and potatoes to the pot. Bring to a boil, reduce heat, cover, and simmer until tender, 20 to 25 minutes.
- Stir in the watercress leaves and cook until just wilted.
- Purée and return to a clean pot.
- Stir in the milk and heat slowly over medium-low heat, stirring frequently.
- Add salt and pepper.
- Garnish with watercress sprigs.

4 to 6 servings

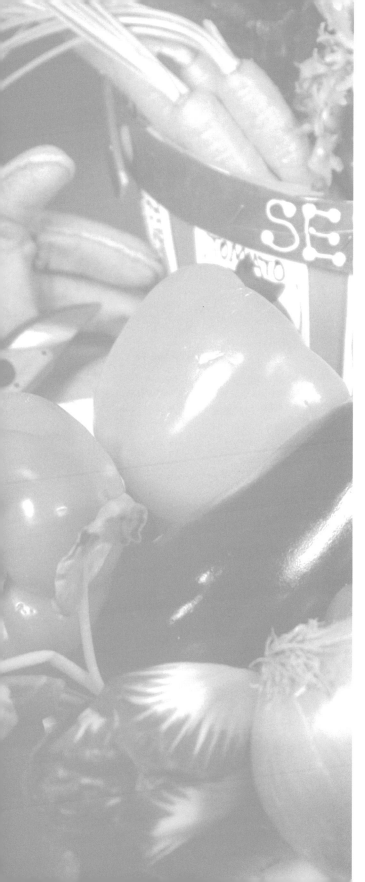

Small Vegetable Dishes

These are the dishes everyone knows how to make, but these are the low-fat versions.

Professional chefs disdain the "dreaded triangle," that is, three food items on a plate: vegetable, starch, protein. As a result, dishes are concocted with dazzling appearances—stacks of artfully arranged slabs of meat or fish precariously balanced on arrays of vegetables or pastry shells and usually floating on a sea of brightly colored liquid, often dotted with individual blobs. These creations are usually impossible to eat in a dignified manner and often run the risk of gracing the diner's lap.

Simplicity should govern the efforts of the dedicated, skilled home cook. Food can dazzle with bright color and artful arrangement on beautiful plates without the frantic quest for originality exhibited by the rock stars of culinary fame!

Artichoke Hearts Sautéed With Wine

A simple-to-prepare dish that promises subtle flavors.

6 large, fresh artichoke hearts, cooked
4 large garlic cloves, minced
1 teaspoon olive oil
1 cup dry, white wine
1 tablespoon fresh thyme, minced
salt
pepper

- Shorten the artichoke stem to 1 inch. Lop off a generous top third of the leaves. Pull off and discard the tough, dark green leaves, leaving the paler, tender inner layers. Bevel the leaves with a sharp knife, leaving a rounded shape resembling the cap of a crimini mushroom. Scoop out the fuzzy, central choke with a melon baller or small spoon. Boil the resulting artichoke hearts in water that has been acidified with the juice and peel of ½ lemon until tender. This should take about 10 minutes or more, depending on the size of the artichokes.

- Cut the cooked artichoke hearts into 8 to 10 pieces.

- Sauté the garlic in the olive oil until it just begins to brown.

- Add the artichoke hearts, wine, and thyme to the pan.

- Simmer for 8 to 10 minutes, basting with the sauce frequently.

- Add salt and pepper.

4 servings

Artichoke Hearts Stuffed With Spinach

Why not? Spinach and artichokes make a colorful accompaniment for spicy tofu or tempeh.

4 large artichokes, fashioned into hearts as in the preceding recipe

8 ounces spinach leaves, washed and chopped fine

2 ounces onion, chopped fine

½ teaspoon olive oil

1 large garlic clove, minced

2 ounces mushrooms, quartered and pulsed in a food processor until chopped fine

salt

pepper

2 large onions, halved lengthwise and sliced

1 teaspoon olive oil

- Boil artichoke hearts for 10 minutes and drain.
- Cook spinach in a small covered pan over medium-low heat, until tender (about 5 minutes). Put the spinach into a sieve and press out all the liquid.
- Sauté the chopped onion in ½ teaspoon olive oil until tender. Add the garlic, briefly stirring.
- Add the mushrooms and cook until they give up all their liquid.
- Combine the spinach-mushroom mixture, salt, and pepper.
- Sauté the 2 sliced onions in 1 teaspoon olive oil over medium heat until well browned, 30 to 40 minutes. Put the browned onion into a flat baking dish.
- Divide the spinach mixture evenly among artichoke hearts and set them on top of the browned onion.
- Cover and bake at 350°F until hot, 25 to 30 minutes.

4 servings

101

Asparagus-Potato Purée

A creamy, pale green meringue-like vegetable side dish that may be combined with colorful, sweet, steamed carrots.

1 pound asparagus, trimmed weight, tough stems removed

1 pound russet potatoes

salt

pepper

- Cut the asparagus into 1-inch pieces and steam until tender, 4 to 8 minutes. Purée and set aside.

- Peel the potatoes and cut them into 1-inch cubes. Steam until tender, about 10 minutes. Put the potatoes through a food mill and combine with the puréed asparagus. Add salt and pepper.

- Turn into a covered casserole and bake at 350°F until very hot, about 25 to 30 minutes.

4 to 6 servings

Steamed Asparagus

Vinegar can add enough flavor interest to asparagus to make it unnecessary to add butter.

1 pound asparagus, washed, tough ends removed

sherry vinegar or balsamic vinegar

- Steam the asparagus until just tender, 4 to 6 minutes.

- Serve hot with sherry vinegar or balsamic vinegar.

4 servings

Asparagus Stir-Fried With Ginger and Soy

Ginger and soy combine to make this asparagus a good mate for soy tofu.

½ teaspoon sesame chili oil

½ teaspoon sesame oil

1 pound asparagus, peeled, trimmed, and cut diagonally into ½-inch-thick pieces

1 tablespoon low-sodium soy sauce

1 teaspoon ginger, minced

2 teaspoons sesame seeds, toasted until golden brown

- Heat the oils in a large skillet over medium heat. Be careful not to heat the oil until it smokes. Stir-fry the asparagus for 2 minutes.
- Add the soy sauce and ginger to the pan. Continue cooking until the asparagus is crisp-tender, 2 to 3 minutes.
- Stir in the sesame seeds.

Variation: Try this with sesame chili oil alone; a generous ½ teaspoon will do.

4 servings

Beets With Orange Juice and Grand Marnier

Try using the beet-peeling technique used in Beet and Orange Salad (page 34). Citrus flavors seem to blend well with the characteristically pungent odor and taste of beets. Small beets are often sweeter and less pungent.

1½ pounds beets, stems cut to 1 inch and scrubbed

½ cup fresh orange juice

3 tablespoons Grand Marnier

zest of 2 oranges

zest of ½ lemon

juice of ½ lemon

salt

- Bake the beets, covered, at 375°F until tender, about 40 to 50 minutes.
- Cool slightly and peel.
- Cut into small cubes.
- Combine the orange juice, Grand Marnier, orange zest, lemon zest, and lemon juice in a pan. Add the beets and stir to combine.
- Cover and heat. Remove from the heat and let stand, covered, for 30 minutes or longer. Reheat and add salt.

Note: Can also be served chilled as a salad.

4 to 6 servings

103

Broccoli Purée

This dish has a plain, wholesome flavor, but it is wholly dependent upon the flavor of the broccoli.

1¾ pounds broccoli, cut into pieces
1 tablespoon plus 1 teaspoon lemon
  juice
1 tablespoon Dijon mustard
salt
pepper

- Steam the broccoli until tender, 6 to 10 minutes.
- Purée the broccoli with the lemon juice and mustard.
- Add salt and pepper.
- Heat in a double boiler.

4 servings

Broccoli Rabe

Try a little bitterness! Young, tender broccoli rabe is less bitter. Choose plants with slender stems, the ends of which, like asparagus spears, should be green and fresh-looking. This vegetable, also known as rapini, is beloved by Italians. Rape seeds are the source of canola oil, which provides omega-3 fatty acids. This cruciferous vegetable once grew wild in California.

1 teaspoon olive oil
3 large garlic cloves, minced
1 bunch broccoli rabe, about 1 pound,
  washed and chopped
1 cup water
salt
pepper

- Heat the olive oil in a pan large enough to hold the broccoli rabe.
- Sauté the garlic briefly and add the broccoli rabe and water. Stir and bring to a boil. Reduce the heat, cover, and simmer until tender (10 to 15 minutes). Add a little more water if necessary.
- Add salt and pepper.

4 servings

Brussels Sprouts With Lemon, Mustard, and Caraway

Citrus and mustard anneal the cabbage-like taste of Brussels sprouts. If you have a mandoline or Benriner (the Japanese version), use it to shred the sprouts.

1 pound trimmed Brussels sprouts, quartered

3½ tablespoons Dijon mustard

1½ tablespoons lemon juice

½ teaspoon caraway seeds

salt

pepper

- Steam the Brussels sprouts until tender, 7 to 8 minutes
- Combine the mustard and lemon juice in a pan large enough to hold the Brussels sprouts. Heat gently.
- Add the cooked Brussels sprouts to the mustard and lemon mixture and stir to coat.
- Stir in the caraway seeds and add salt and pepper.

4 servings

Cabbage and Scallions Sauté

The cabbage can be toasted slightly to add a bit of caramel flavor.

1 teaspoon olive oil

4 cups green cabbage, shredded by hand

1 cup scallions, sliced

salt

- Heat the olive oil in a large pan and sauté the cabbage and scallions until crisp-tender, 8 to 10 minutes.
- Add salt.

2 servings

107

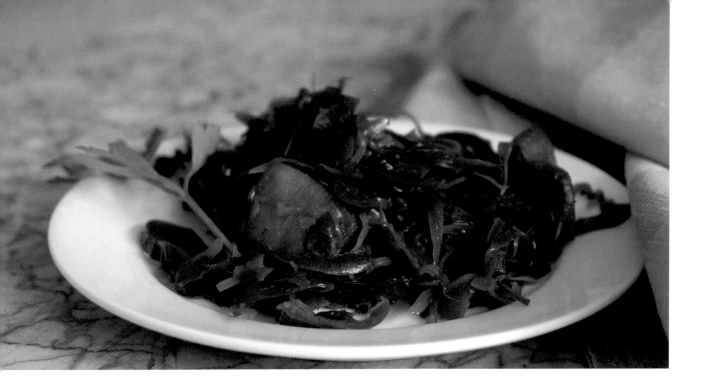

Red Cabbage With Apple

Sweet-sour, spicy flavors transform the cabbage in this dish, making it a succulent delight.

1 onion (about 8 ounces), halved and sliced

1 teaspoon olive oil

¾ pound red cabbage, shredded by hand

1½ pounds Fuji apples, peeled, cored, and sliced; cut the slices in half

1 tablespoon dark brown sugar

1 tablespoon cider vinegar

pinch of ground cloves

⅛ teaspoon cinnamon

pinch of nutmeg

½ cup beer

salt

- Sauté the onion in the olive oil until tender.

- Add the cabbage and sauté for 5 minutes. Cover and simmer for 10 minutes.

- Add the apples, brown sugar, vinegar, cloves, cinnamon, nutmeg, and beer. Simmer, covered, for 20 minutes or until tender.

- Add salt.

4 to 6 servings

Glazed Carrots

Coating carrots with sweetness complements the native sweetness of the carrots themselves.

3 tablespoons brandy

3 tablespoons dark brown sugar, packed

3 tablespoons orange juice

1¼ pounds carrots, peeled and sliced

salt

zest of 1 orange

- Combine the brandy, brown sugar, and orange juice in a pan and simmer gently until the sauce begins to thicken, 4 to 5 minutes.
- Steam the carrots until tender, 10 to 12 minutes, and add to the sauce. Add salt and the orange zest. Simmer for 2 to 3 minutes.

4 servings

Curried Cauliflower Purée

Cauliflower is bland. Curry flavor, especially in this purée, lifts it to a higher level.

1 pound plus 10 ounces cauliflower, cut into small pieces

4 tablespoons mild chutney

¾ teaspoon or more curry powder

salt

- Steam the cauliflower until tender, 8 to 10 minutes, and purée with the chutney and curry powder.
- Add salt.
- Heat in a double boiler.

4 servings

109

Cauliflower-Pea Purée

The flavor of fresh, seasonal English peas: sweet blends with the taste of cauliflower and onions, yielding a mild but delicious combination.

1 pound cauliflower, cut into flowerets
1 onion (about 8 ounces), sliced
1 teaspoon olive oil
2 cups fresh peas
¼ cup nonfat milk
salt
pepper

- Steam the cauliflower until tender, 6 to 10 minutes.
- Sauté the onion in the olive oil until tender.
- Boil the peas until tender, 3 to 10 minutes, and drain.
- Purée the cauliflower, onion, peas, and milk until smooth.
- Add salt and pepper.
- Heat in a double boiler.

4 to 6 servings

Cauliflower With Tomatoes

The tangy, sweet-tart flavor of tomatoes—fresh tomatoes—does add some punch to the mildness of cauliflower.

1 large onion (about 1 pound), halved lengthwise and sliced thin

1 teaspoon olive oil

2 large garlic cloves, minced

2 pounds tomatoes, peeled and chopped

1 pound cauliflower flowerets

4 teaspoons fresh oregano, chopped

salt

pepper

- Sauté the onion in the olive oil until tender. Add the garlic, briefly stirring.
- Add the tomatoes to the pot and simmer until the sauce has thickened, 20 to 30 minutes.
- Add the cauliflower and oregano to the tomatoes. Simmer, uncovered, until tender (about 10 to 12 minutes).
- Add salt and pepper.

4 servings

Cherry Tomato Sauté

Here is a condiment-like addition to a savory slice of tofu.

1 pound small cherry tomatoes

1 teaspoon olive oil

- Pierce the skin of each tomato with a fork.
- Heat the olive oil in a nonstick skillet over medium heat.
- Sauté the tomatoes until hot, about 3 minutes.
- Do not overcook.

4 servings

111

Colcannon

This dish is often described as an Irish peasant concoction. The lack of fat in this version would make this a dish for slender Irish peasants.

1½ pounds russet potatoes, peeled and cut into ½-inch cubes

5 whole, large garlic cloves, peeled

¾ to 1 cup nonfat milk

1 teaspoon salt

pepper

1 teaspoon olive oil

6 cups (about 1 pound) green cabbage or kale, shredded by hand

1 bunch scallions, including the green tops, sliced thin, about 1 cup

paprika

- Steam the potatoes and garlic until very tender, about 10 minutes.
- Put the potatoes and garlic through a food mill into a pan.
- Stir in some of the milk with the salt and pepper. Cover the pan and heat the potatoes, stirring often, 10 to 12 minutes. Add more milk if necessary to keep the potatoes creamy while heating.
- While the potatoes are heating, heat the olive oil in a large pan and sauté the cabbage or kale with the scallions until crisp-tender, about 8 to 10 minutes.
- Stir the cabbage or kale and scallions into the heated potatoes and heat 3 to 4 minutes.
- Sprinkle each serving lightly with paprika.

4 servings

Corn and Tomatoes

Corn and tomatoes are a matchless combination, repeated often in Mexican cooking.

10 ounces tomatoes, peeled and chopped

4 ears corn, kernels cut from the cob (3 to 3½ cups)

salt

pepper

- Cook the tomatoes until soft, about 6 minutes.
- Add the corn to the pot, cover, and cook gently until the corn is crisp-tender, about 8 minutes.
- Add salt and pepper.

4 servings

Corn-Tomato-Zucchini–Red Pepper Sauté

Care is needed to avoid overcooking the zucchini, which should be crisp-tender, not a gelatinous lump.

4 ounces onion, chopped

1 teaspoon olive oil

2 ears of corn, kernels cut from the cob

1 large tomato, peeled and chopped

1 red pepper, seeded and sliced

1 teaspoon fresh thyme, chopped

12 ounces zucchini, cut into ½-inch cubes

salt

pepper

- Sauté the onion in the olive oil until tender.
- Add the corn, tomato, red pepper, and thyme. Cook gently, covered, for 5 minutes.
- Add the zucchini and continue cooking, covered, for 5 minutes or until the zucchini is crisp-tender.
- Add salt and pepper.

4 servings

113

Eggplant and Tomatoes With Currants

Adding currants, cumin, and cinnamon turns this eggplant combination into an unusually savory blend.

2 teaspoons garlic, minced

1 teaspoon olive oil

14 ounces Roma tomatoes, peeled and chopped

10 ounces slender eggplant, cut into small pieces

¼ teaspoon cinnamon

¼ teaspoon ground cumin

¼ cup currants

salt

pepper

- Sauté the garlic in the olive oil briefly.
- Add the tomatoes and cook, uncovered, for 20 minutes.
- Add the eggplant, cinnamon, and cumin. Cook, covered, for 5 minutes.
- Add the currants and continue cooking until the eggplant is done, about 10 more minutes.
- Add salt and pepper.

3 to 4 servings

Eggplant, Tomatoes, and Herbs

Try adding stems of fresh oregano and thyme, removing them, of course, before serving. Another herb, basil—especially an exotic variety such as Thai basil or the African variety—certainly adds rich flavor to an eggplant dish.

8 ounces onion, chopped

1 teaspoon olive oil

4 garlic cloves, minced

1½ pounds Roma tomatoes, peeled and chopped

2 teaspoons fresh oregano, chopped

1 teaspoon fresh thyme, chopped

1 pound slender or round eggplant, cut into small cubes

salt

pepper

- Sauté the onion in the olive oil until soft. Add the garlic, briefly stirring.
- Add the tomatoes and herbs to the pot and simmer for 15 minutes.
- Add the cubed eggplant to the tomatoes, cover, and simmer until the eggplant is tender, 25 to 30 minutes. If the tomatoes are not juicy, it may be necessary to add a little water to cook the eggplant.
- Add salt and pepper.

4 servings

Fava Beans

Also known as broad beans, fava beans *are* broad, perhaps 8 inches long. All of the other "beans" are New World plants discovered in the Americas and returned to Europe for cultivation. Broad beans have a slightly nutty flavor. Here, they are joined to the mild flavors of lettuce and the moderated zing of garlic sautéed in wine.

3 pounds fava beans

3 ounces onion, chopped

1 teaspoon olive oil

2 large garlic cloves, minced

2 large leaf lettuce leaves, chopped

½ cup dry, white wine

salt

pepper

- Shell the fava beans and drop them into boiling water for 30 seconds. Drain and rinse with cold water. Make a small slit in one end of the bean skin and slip out the bean.

- In a small pan, sauté the onion in the olive oil until soft. Add the garlic, briefly stirring.

- Add the lettuce leaves and fava beans to the pot. Cook gently, covered, over low heat for 10 minutes, stirring several times.

- Add the wine and simmer, covered, for 10 minutes or until the beans are tender.

- Add salt and pepper.

4 servings

Fries

Immerse the potato sticks in chilled water for a short time before coating them with flavor.

1 teaspoon chili powder

½ teaspoon garlic powder

¼ teaspoon paprika

¼ teaspoon ground cumin

⅛ teaspoon turmeric

⅛ teaspoon black pepper

salt

¼ cup Vegetable Broth (page 58)

2 large russet potatoes, scrubbed, cut into ½-inch sticks and immersed in cold water

- Mix the chili powder, garlic powder, paprika, cumin, turmeric, pepper, and salt.
- Toss the potatoes with the broth; drain.
- Sprinkle the dry mixture gradually on the potatoes, stirring to coat them evenly.
- Arrange the coated potatoes on 2 baking sheets in a single layer.
- Bake in a preheated 450°F oven for 30 to 40 minutes until crisp. Loosen the potatoes with a spatula at 8 minutes to prevent sticking. Repeat twice during the cooking time.
- Serve with Homemade Catsup (page 226).

2 servings

Green Beans and Tomatoes

Another almost insultingly simple combination. Vegetables don't have to be served in elaborate uniforms. Simplicity is often preferable and highlights the flavors of the fresh ingredients themselves.

8 ounces onion, chopped

1 teaspoon olive oil

3 large garlic cloves, minced

1 pound tomatoes, peeled and chopped

1 pound green beans or haricots verts, trimmed and broken into 1-inch lengths

salt

pepper

- Sauté the onions in the olive oil until tender. Add the garlic, briefly stirring.
- Add the tomatoes and cook over medium heat for 15 minutes.
- Boil the beans until crisp-tender, 3 to 5 minutes. Drain and add to the tomatoes.
- Simmer until beans are tender, 5 to 10 minutes.
- Add salt and pepper.

4 to 6 servings

Green Beans and Mushrooms

Try trumpet or oyster mushrooms.

8 ounces mushrooms, sliced

1 pound green beans, trimmed and broken into 2-inch lengths

salt

pepper

- Sauté the mushrooms in a skillet until tender and a small amount of their liquid remains.
- Boil the beans until tender, 6 to 12 minutes. Drain the beans and add them to the mushrooms.
- Add salt and pepper.
- Cover the skillet and heat for 2 to 3 minutes.

4 servings

Green Beans With Sesame Chili Oil

Be sure to use the toasted variety of hot sesame oil. It really has much more sesame flavor, the difference between sesame seeds and toasted seeds, a big boost in flavor and aroma.

1 pound green beans, ends removed, broken into 2-inch lengths

1 teaspoon sesame chili oil

½ teaspoon low-sodium soy sauce

salt

- Boil the beans until tender, 5 to 10 minutes.
- Heat the oil gently in pan. Be careful to avoid burning the oil; it burns easily.
- Add the beans to the oil along with the soy sauce and salt. Sauté briefly until heated.

2 servings

Green Bean–Potato Purée

Potatoes can be a mild-tasting delight paired with the green taste of fresh green beans. Choose tender, seasonal Blue Lake beans, which are best from May through August. Stale, tough beans will taste like cardboard. Homegrown beans just picked from the bush will delight.

1 pound green beans, trimmed and broken into 2-inch lengths

1 pound peeled russet potatoes, cut into 1-inch cubes

⅛ teaspoon freshly grated nutmeg

salt

pepper

- Boil the beans until tender, about 6 minutes. Drain and purée.
- Steam the potatoes until tender, 10 to 12 minutes. Put the potatoes through a food mill and mix with the puréed beans.
- Add the nutmeg, salt, and pepper.
- Bake, covered, at 350°F until hot, about 25 minutes.

4 servings

119

Peas and Mushrooms

Try a different mushroom every time you do this dish: porcini, shiitake, chanterelle, trumpet, even crimini.

6 ounces mushrooms, sliced thin

3 cups fresh peas

salt

pepper

- Sauté the mushrooms in a medium skillet until tender and a small amount of liquid remains, 5 to 6 minutes.
- Boil the peas until tender, 3 to 10 minutes, and drain. Add the peas to the mushrooms with salt and pepper.
- Cover the skillet and heat for 2 to 3 minutes.

4 to 6 servings

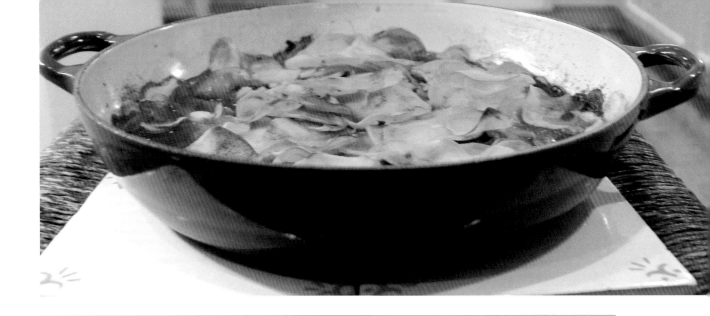

Potato Casserole

Try this dish with nonfat milk instead of broth, but use more seasoning: savory, epazote, thyme, even a bit of cayenne.

1 pound onion, chopped

1 teaspoon olive oil

2 pounds russet potatoes, peeled and sliced 2 mm (about 7/64 inch) thick in a food processor

½ teaspoon dried rosemary, crumbled

salt

pepper

2¼ cups Vegetable Broth (page 58)

- Sauté the onion in the olive oil until well browned.
- Layer the potatoes, onion, and rosemary in a shallow, heavy, 3-quart cast-iron or ceramic baking dish, sprinkling each layer with salt and pepper.
- Pour 1¼ cups broth over the potatoes.
- Bake, uncovered, at 350°F, basting often. Add the remaining broth gradually as the sauce thickens. Bake until done, 1 to 1¼ hours.

4 to 6 servings

Potatoes—Mashed With Garlic, or With Garlic and Basil

For a change, experiment with other potatoes, perhaps Yukon Golds or new potatoes.

1½ pounds russet potatoes, peeled and cut into ½-inch cubes

5 large, whole garlic cloves, peeled

¾ to 1 cup nonfat milk

1 teaspoon salt

pepper

- Steam the potatoes and garlic together until very tender, about 12 minutes.
- Put the potatoes and garlic through a food mill into a heavy pan with a lid.
- Stir in ½ cup milk, 1 teaspoon salt, and pepper. Cover the pan and heat over medium-low heat, stirring often until hot, 12 to 14 minutes.
- Gradually stir in more milk as necessary to keep potatoes creamy while heating.

Variation: Stir 2 teaspoons fresh, minced basil into the potatoes while heating.

3 to 4 servings

Potatoes With Paprika

This recipe yields plump, flavorful potato wedges with no added fat. Use Hungarian paprika if you like, but if you use the smoky or hot varieties, try mixing them with an equal amount of your usual paprika.

2 large russet potatoes, 1½ pounds, scrubbed

salt

pepper

paprika

- Halve the potatoes lengthwise. Place the cut sides down and halve again lengthwise. Cut each quarter into 2 equal wedges. Immerse the potato wedges in cold water for about 15 minutes.
- Sprinkle the cut surfaces with salt and pepper, then sprinkle generously with paprika.
- Place the potato wedges in a single layer in a 2-inch-deep pan.
- Bake at 450°F for 35 to 40 minutes until tender.
- Serve with catsup.

3 to 4 servings

Potatoes Baked in a Tomato Sauce

The success of this delightful dish depends on persistent and thorough mixing of the first 6 ingredients with the potatoes. Mix while separating the potato slices, which stubbornly try to stick together. The end result is worth the effort. Use Greek or Syrian oregano if you can find it.

8 ounces red pepper, seeded and sliced

1½ teaspoons olive oil

3 large garlic cloves, minced

12 ounces mixed vegetable juice

2 tablespoons fresh oregano, chopped

8 ounces tomatoes, peeled and chopped

1½ pounds russet potatoes, peeled and sliced 2 mm (about 7/64 inch) thick in a food processor

salt

pepper

- Sauté the red pepper in the olive oil until crisp-tender, about 10 minutes. Add the garlic, briefly stirring. Transfer to a large bowl.
- Add the mixed vegetable juice, oregano, and tomatoes to the bowl and combine.
- Add the potatoes, salt, and pepper. Mix, and be sure the potatoes are separated and coated with liquid.
- Transfer to a 10-inch-square baking dish, 2½ inches deep. A 2-quart, 2-inch-deep pan will do.
- Bake, covered, in a 350°F oven until tender.

4 servings

Potatoes and Wine

For this dish, you must assume the identity of a Basque herdsman in northern Spain. You have only a 6-inch knife on your belt. Cut the onion into chunks and the potato into roughly similar pieces. Roast the onions in the bottom of a large metal pot over a blazing wood fire, splashing the local, robust wine over the potatoes, turning them blue-red.

5 ounces onion, cut into 1-inch cubes

1 teaspoon olive oil

2 pounds russet potatoes, peeled and cut into 1-inch cubes

1 cup dry, red wine

1 bay leaf

salt

pepper

- Sauté the onion in the olive oil until brown, about 15 minutes.
- Add the potatoes, wine, and bay leaf. Simmer, covered, until just soft (about 20 minutes), stirring often.
- Add salt and pepper.

4 servings

Red Potatoes Roasted With Garlic or Onion

A bit of garlic or onion adds interest.

1½ pounds red potatoes, cut into ½-inch slices

5 large garlic cloves, peeled and halved lengthwise, and/or 1 medium onion, sliced thin

1 teaspoon olive oil

salt and pepper

- Combine all the ingredients in a bowl just large enough to contain them, then transfer to a flat baking dish in a single layer.
- Bake, uncovered, at 400°F for 25 to 35 minutes or until tender.
- Stir after 10 minutes and several more times during baking.

Variation: Use an 8-ounce onion, roughly sliced, instead of the garlic. An equivalent amount of sliced shallots will also do. About ½ teaspoon crushed rosemary can be added in either case.

4 servings

127

Turnips, Carrots, and Onions—Roasted

Root vegetables roasted together blend well.

1 teaspoon olive oil

8 ounces turnips, peeled and cut into 1-inch cubes

14 ounces carrots, peeled and cut into 1-inch cubes

8 ounces boiling onions, peeled

salt

pepper

- Spray or wipe the olive oil on a baking dish large enough to hold the vegetables.
- Add the vegetables to the dish and add salt and pepper. Mix to coat the vegetables with the olive oil.
- Cover and bake at 400°F until the vegetables are tender, 20 to 30 minutes.

4 servings

Zucchini With Fresh Tomato Sauce

Don't overcook the zucchini; they should be just edging toward softness.

2 pounds tomatoes, peeled and chopped

salt

pepper

1 pound zucchini, halved lengthwise and sliced ¼ inch thick

2 tablespoons fresh oregano, chopped

- Cook the tomatoes gently, uncovered, until soft and the liquid has evaporated, about 1 hour.
- Purée and add salt and pepper. Heat, uncovered.
- Bake the zucchini slices at 325°F for 4 minutes.
- Serve topped with the heated sauce and sprinkle with the chopped oregano.

4 servings

142

Stuffed Zucchini With Tomato Sauce

Whole-grain bulgur and mushrooms with a trifle of spice in little zucchini boats, hot from the oven, are most appealing.

4 zucchini, 6 inches long

½ cup shallots, chopped

2 ounces mushrooms, chopped fine

1 teaspoon olive oil

½ cup boiling water

generous ¼ cup bulgur, uncooked

1 teaspoon fresh oregano, chopped

2 tablespoons double-concentrated Italian tomato paste (comes in a tube)

salt

pepper

Sauce:

1 pound tomatoes, peeled and chopped

2 teaspoons fresh oregano, chopped

salt

- Begin by preparing the sauce. Combine the tomatoes and oregano in a small pot. Bring to a boil, reduce heat, and simmer until thick (about 30 minutes). Purée and return to the pan.

- Add salt and set aside.

- Cut the ends from the zucchini and cut them in half lengthwise. Carefully scoop out the flesh with a melon baller, leaving a ¼-inch shell.

- Pulse the zucchini flesh in a food processor to chop fine.

- Sauté the shallots, mushrooms, and chopped zucchini in the olive oil until tender and transfer to a bowl.

- Pour the boiling water over the bulgur. Cover and let stand for 15 minutes. Drain.

- Combine the zucchini mixture, bulgur, oregano, and tomato paste.

- Add salt and pepper.

- Divide the zucchini mixture evenly among the shells. Place in a baking dish or pan. Cover and bake at 350°F until hot, 25 to 30 minutes.

- Heat the tomato sauce and serve with the zucchini.

4 servings

143

Zucchini, Tomatoes, and Shallots With Oregano

Shallots zip up the zucchini flavor.

1 pound zucchini, halved lengthwise
   and sliced

1 large tomato, peeled and chopped

½ cup shallots, chopped

2 large garlic cloves, minced

1 tablespoon lemon juice

1 tablespoon fresh oregano, chopped

2 tablespoons parsley, chopped

salt

pepper

- Cook the zucchini, tomato, shallots, and garlic, covered, over low heat in a 10-inch sauté pan until the zucchini is barely tender, 10 to 15 minutes, stirring occasionally.
- Add the lemon juice, oregano, parsley, salt, and pepper.
- Heat for 2 to 3 minutes and serve.

4 servings

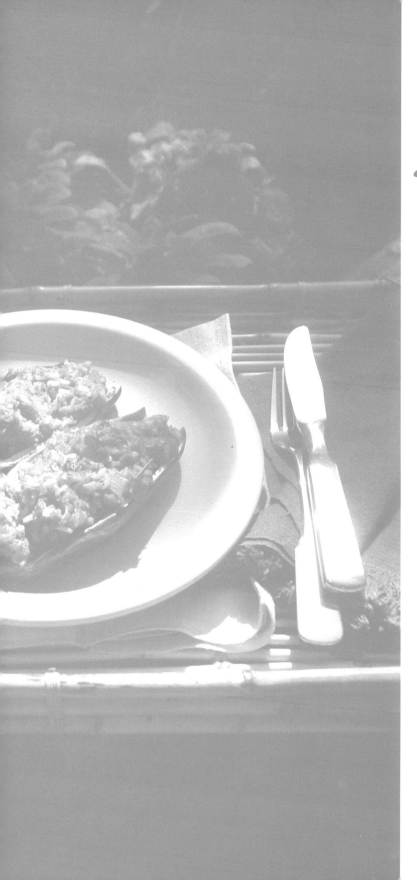

Main
Dishes

Beer-Simmered Beans

Beer's flavor complements the beans and tomatoes in this combination, adding flavor without fat.

1 pound pinto beans, sorted and rinsed

1 small onion (roughly 8 ounces), chopped

1 teaspoon olive oil

4 large garlic cloves, minced

12 ounces Heineken beer or a malty beer

4 cups Vegetable Broth (page 58)

1 8-ounce can tomato sauce

1½ teaspoons crushed red pepper flakes

1 tablespoon fresh oregano, chopped

2 teaspoons ground cumin

3 tablespoons double-concentrated Italian tomato paste (comes in a tube)

1 tablespoon low-sodium soy sauce

salt

cilantro, coarsely chopped

- Boil the beans in a large quantity of water for 2 minutes. Remove from heat, cover, and let stand for 1 hour. Drain and rinse.

- Sauté the onion in the olive oil until soft. Add the garlic, briefly stirring.

- Add the drained beans, beer, vegetable broth, tomato sauce, red pepper flakes, oregano, and cumin to the pot.

- Bring to a boil, reduce the heat, and simmer, partially covered, stirring occasionally until tender, 1¾ to 2 hours. Add a small quantity of boiling water as needed during the cooking to keep the beans just covered with liquid.

- Stir in the tomato paste and soy sauce.

- Add salt.

- Stir in the cilantro just before serving.

6 servings

Black Beans With Rice

Black beans have a rich, almost pungent flavor. They are cooked in this dish so enough of the thickened sauce anoints the rice.

1 pound black beans, sorted and rinsed
1 pound onion, chopped
4 large garlic cloves, minced
1 bay leaf
1¼ teaspoons dry oregano
1½ teaspoons crushed red pepper flakes
⅓ cup parsley, chopped
3 cups Vegetable Broth (page 58)
7 cups water
1 teaspoon salt
rice
cilantro for garnish

- Combine the black beans, onion, garlic, bay leaf, oregano, pepper flakes, parsley, broth, water, and salt in a pot. Bring to a boil, reduce heat, and simmer, uncovered, until the beans are tender and the sauce is thick, 1¾ to 2 hours. Add additional water, if necessary, to keep the beans just covered.
- Serve with cooked rice and garnish with cilantro.

6 servings

Beans on Toast

Putting beans on toast, instead of on rice, makes this an almost festive dish—and one you could enjoy at breakfast.

1½ cups red kidney beans, sorted and rinsed

1 teaspoon salt

12 ounces onion, chopped

1½ cups green bell pepper, chopped

1 teaspoon olive oil

4 garlic cloves, minced

2½ cups tomato sauce

¾ cup dry, red wine

2½ teaspoons chili powder

1 teaspoon dark molasses

1 tablespoon French's mustard

3 teaspoons horseradish

salt

pepper

6 slices whole-grain bread, toasted

6 medium tomatoes, sliced and baked at 350°F for 5 to 7 minutes or until hot

- Bring the beans and the 1 teaspoon salt to a boil in enough water to cover by several inches. Reduce the heat and cook gently, uncovered, until done, about 1 hour. Drain the beans, rinse with cold water, and set aside.

- Sauté the onion and the green bell pepper in the olive oil until soft. Add the garlic, briefly stirring.

- Add the tomato sauce, wine, chili powder, molasses, mustard, horseradish, and the cooked beans to the pot. Simmer for 20 minutes.

- Add salt and pepper.

- Serve the beans on top of the toasted bread.

- Top with the tomato slices.

6 servings

Garbanzo Beans With Couscous

Couscous is a whole-wheat pasta, a form of grain that originated in North Africa. It is a light rice substitute, contrastingly fluffy in texture and very easily prepared. Its flavor blends well with the mild taste of garbanzo beans.

8 ounces onion, chopped

9 ounces red bell pepper, seeded and chopped coarse

1 teaspoon olive oil

2 garlic cloves, minced

1 pound tomatoes, peeled and chopped

1½ teaspoons curry powder

¼ teaspoon ground cumin

¼ teaspoon ground coriander

1 16-ounce can garbanzo beans, drained and rinsed

salt

pepper

1½ cups whole-wheat couscous, uncooked

¾ cup Vegetable Broth (page 58)

- Sauté the onion and the red bell pepper in the olive oil until tender.
- Add the garlic, briefly stirring.
- Add the tomatoes, curry powder, cumin, and coriander to the pot. Simmer rapidly for 10 minutes, uncovered.
- Add the beans and simmer, covered, for 10 minutes.
- Add salt and pepper.
- Bring the broth to a boil and stir the couscous into the boiling broth. Remove from the heat, cover, and let stand for 5 minutes. Stir to fluff.
- Serve the beans over the couscous.

3 servings

Garbanzo Beans and Vegetables

More beans and couscous, but this iteration with potatoes and zucchini.

8 ounces onion, chopped

1 cup green bell pepper, chopped

1 cup red bell pepper, chopped

1 teaspoon olive oil

1½ teaspoons cinnamon

1 teaspoon ground coriander

1 pound sweet potatoes, peeled and cut into ½-inch cubes

1½ pounds tomatoes, peeled and chopped

1 16-ounce can low-salt garbanzo beans, drained and rinsed

¼ cup water

¼ teaspoon crushed red pepper flakes

¾ teaspoon salt

4 ounces zucchini, cut into ½-inch cubes

1½ cups water

½ teaspoons salt

1 cup couscous

- Sauté the onion and bell peppers in the olive oil until soft.
- Add the cinnamon and coriander. Cook briefly, stirring.
- Add the sweet potatoes and cook for 2 minutes, stirring.
- Add the tomatoes, garbanzo beans, ¼ cup water, pepper flakes, and ¾ teaspoon salt to the pot. Cook gently, covered, for 15 minutes.
- Add the zucchini and continue cooking, covered, until the sweet potatoes are tender (10 to 15 minutes).
- Bring the 1½ cups water and ½ teaspoon salt to a boil. Stir in the couscous and remove from heat. Cover and let stand for 5 minutes. Stir with a fork and serve with the vegetables.

6 servings

Mexican Beans

This is a bean combination with high flavor. Serve it with tortillas and a salad, and perhaps pico de gallo.

Beans:

1 small onion (about 8 ounces), chopped

1 teaspoon olive oil

1 pound pinto beans, sorted and rinsed

salt

Beans:

- Sauté the onion in the olive oil until tender.
- Add the beans, salt, and enough water to cover by several inches. Bring to a boil, reduce heat, and simmer until the beans are tender, about 1½ hours. Add water, if necessary, to keep the beans covered. Drain and set aside.

Sauce:

1 pound onion, chopped

1 teaspoon olive oil

5 large garlic cloves, minced

2 tablespoons chili powder

1 teaspoon ground cumin

2 pounds tomatoes, peeled and chopped

¼ teaspoon crushed red pepper flakes

¾ cup red bell pepper, chopped

¾ cup green bell pepper, chopped

salt

Sauce:

- Sauté the onion in the olive oil until tender. Add the garlic, briefly stirring.
- Add the chili powder and cumin to the pan and sauté for 1 minute.
- Add the tomatoes and red pepper flakes to the pan. Cook until the tomatoes begin to soften, 5 to 10 minutes.
- Add the red and green bell pepper and cook for 2 to 3 minutes.
- Add the beans and cook slowly, covered, for 30 minutes.
- Add salt.

6 to 8 servings

151

Refried Beans

These very plain beans are a good foil for a spicy vegetable like curried tomatoes or even spinach with browned onion. Jazz them up, if you wish, by adding a jalapeño chili or some spicy fried eggs. (A *rare* egg—4.5 grams of fat—is a minor dietary lapse.)

¾ pound pinto beans, sorted and rinsed
12 ounces onion, chopped
¼ teaspoon salt

- Combine the beans, onion, and salt in a large pot.
- Add water to cover by several inches.
- Bring to a boil, reduce heat, and simmer until beans are soft, 1½ to 1¾ hours. Add additional hot water, if necessary, to keep the beans just covered while cooking. Stir occasionally to prevent sticking.
- Purée the beans and add more salt.
- Heat the beans slowly in a heavy pan, stirring often. If the beans seem too thick, add a little water.

4 to 6 servings

Bean and Rice Casserole

Corn and beans are perfect complements.

1 pound onion, chopped

1 teaspoon olive oil

5 large garlic cloves, minced (2 tablespoons)

1 pound tomatoes, peeled and chopped

1 cup red bell pepper, chopped

1½ cups rice

2²/₃ cups Vegetable Broth (page 58)

2 16-ounce cans low-sodium garbanzo beans, drained and rinsed

2 ears corn, kernels cut from the cob

1 tablespoon fresh oregano (or 1 teaspoon dried oregano)

¼ teaspoon crushed red pepper flakes

1 teaspoon salt

pepper

- Sauté the onion in the olive oil until tender. Add the garlic, briefly stirring.
- Add the tomatoes and cook for 10 minutes.
- Add the red bell pepper and cook for 2 minutes.
- Add the remaining ingredients and bring to a boil, stirring often.
- Turn into a baking dish, cover, and bake at 400°F for 25 minutes.

8 servings

Indian Vegetarian Patties/Croquettes

Classic Indian pastries, aloo samosas, are pastry wrappers that are often filled with cooked potatoes, peas, and even puréed pomegranate seeds, then deep-fried. The humble patties in this recipe can be browned and flavorful with the use of minimal fat. The rather preliminary spices suggested can be adjusted on further trials by using sambhar curry powder together with more ginger, cumin, turmeric, and perhaps the more complex and nuanced heat of small red Indian chilis when they can be paired with some cooling yogurt-based raita.

1 cup fresh corn (about 1 ear)

½ cup English peas, cooked

½ cup carrot, grated fine, about 2 ounces

8 ounces russet potato, peeled and grated fine

3 large spinach leaves, chopped fine, about 1 cup (chopped before measuring and loosely packed)

4 ounces onion, chopped fine

⅓ cup cilantro, chopped fine

2 teaspoons garlic, minced (a small clove)

1 teaspoon curry powder

¼ teaspoon red pepper flakes

2 teaspoons ginger, minced

1 teaspoon ground cumin

½ teaspoon turmeric

6 tablespoons flour

2 egg whites, beaten

salt

1 to 2 teaspoons olive oil

- Cook the corn on the cob using Craig Claiborne's method: Put the corn in a pot of boiling water sufficient to cover. When the water boils again, cover the pot, remove from heat, and let stand 5 minutes. Stand the ear at attention when it has cooled a bit, and cut the kernels from the cob.

- Boil the peas until just tender, a process that could take 4 to 10-plus minutes.

- Combine all of the ingredients except the olive oil and pulse them in a food processor just until the constituents are coarsely chopped. Form the ingredients into patties or croquette shapes and chill them until firm, about 4 hours. Sauté the patties in a nonstick pan evenly misted with 1 to 2 teaspoons olive oil until they are browned on both sides, about 10 minutes. Cook them over a moderate flame so the vegetables are heated through.

About 12 makes for a size easily sautéed.

Zucchini Burgers

Small, youthful zucchini work best. The best, indeed, are homegrown squashes. The wheat germ and egg whites add about 7 grams of protein to each burger.

2 cups zucchini, about 1¼ pounds, grated fine by hand; measure after squeezing out as much liquid as possible

¾ cup wheat germ

1 large garlic clove, minced

3 ounces onion, minced

1½ cups mushrooms, chopped fine

¼ teaspoon dry thyme

¼ teaspoon dry oregano

2 egg whites

1½ teaspoons salt

pepper

1½ teaspoons olive oil

- Just before cooking, combine all the ingredients except the olive oil.
- Shape into 8 burgers.
- Heat the olive oil in a nonstick pan and cook the burgers over medium-low heat until golden brown, about 7 minutes per side, turning once.
- Serve with plain, nonfat yogurt.
- Burgers can also be served in pita bread with sprouts, tomato, Maui onion, pickles, and mustard sauce: 1 cup plain, nonfat yogurt and 2 tablespoons mustard, whisked together.

8 burgers

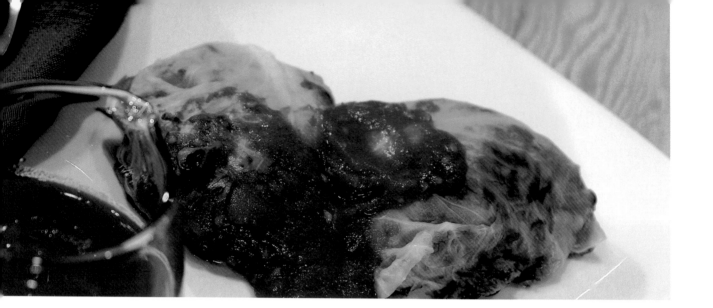

Cabbage Rolls Stuffed With a Savory Rice and Mushroom Mixture

Do wear rubber gloves, preferably the thin, surgical type, when you are dealing with the cabbage to avoid scalding your hands. These little packages look and taste impressive. Handle them carefully, and they shouldn't need to be secured with kitchen string.

4 pounds tomatoes, peeled and chopped

½ teaspoon salt

⅔ cup brown rice, uncooked

8 ounces onion, chopped

1 teaspoon olive oil

2 or 3 large garlic cloves, minced

8 ounces mushrooms, chopped

1½ teaspoons dried oregano

salt

pepper

1 green cabbage—choose a large head

- Cook the tomatoes, uncovered, until soft and no longer watery (about 45 minutes). Add salt. Purée. Set ½ cup purée aside and put a thin layer of the purée into a 10-inch-square baking dish.

- Boil the brown rice gently for 30 minutes in enough water to cover generously. Drain and set aside.

- Sauté the onion in the olive oil until soft. Add the garlic, briefly stirring. Add the mushrooms and continue cooking until tender and the liquid has just evaporated.

(continued)

- Combine the mushroom mixture in a bowl with the cooked rice, ½ cup tomato purée, oregano, salt, and pepper. Flatten the mixture in the bottom of the bowl and score the surface into 8 equal parts.

- Remove the discolored outer cabbage leaves, if necessary, and discard them. Core the cabbage and plunge it whole into boiling water for several minutes until the leaves begin to come away from the head. The cabbage will float. Spin it and encourage it to remain submerged. Ease cabbage out of the boiling water with a slotted spoon and your gloved hand. Carefully remove 8 leaves. Drop the leaves into boiling water, 2 at a time for about 2 minutes, until just tender. Drop the leaves into ice water to chill, and gently blot dry.

- Cut a V-shaped wedge about 1 inch long from the base of each leaf. Put ⅛ of the rice mixture on the base of each leaf. Fold the stem end of the leaf over the rice mixture, folding the leaf sides inward, enclosing the stuffing. Continue rolling toward the leaf tip to form a compact roll. You may need to turn the leaf packages facedown when you place the rolls on top of the tomato purée in the baking dish.

- Bake, covered, at 350°F until hot, 40 minutes.

- Heat the remaining tomato purée in a pot and serve with the cabbage rolls.

8 cabbage rolls

Kugel

This traditional pudding-like dish makes a good, bland counterpart for a spicy tempeh or tofu dish.

1 small onion (roughly 8 ounces)
2¼ to 2½ pounds russet potatoes
2 teaspoons olive oil
1 egg, beaten
¾ teaspoon salt
pepper

Dressing:
4 teaspoons horseradish
1½ cups plain, nonfat yogurt

- Heat the oven to 350°F.
- Peel the onion and grate it in a food processor fitted with a medium grating disc.
- Peel the potatoes and grate them in a food processor fitted with a medium grating disc.
- Heat the olive oil in a shallow 10- by 10-inch baking dish in the oven for 4 to 10 minutes. Tilt the pan to coat the bottom evenly.
- Combine the grated onion and potatoes, egg, salt, and pepper in a bowl.
- Put the mixture into the baking dish with heated oil and distribute evenly.
- Bake, uncovered, for 60 to 65 minutes until browned and crisp around the edges.
- Whisk together the horseradish and yogurt. Serve with the kugel.

4 to 6 servings

Corn-Topped Beans

This dish looks especially appetizing when it comes steaming-hot from the oven.

Beans:

1 cup red kidney beans, sorted and rinsed

¾ teaspoon salt

12 ounces onion, chopped

1½ cups green bell pepper, chopped

1 teaspoon olive oil

3 large garlic cloves, minced

2 pounds tomatoes, peeled and chopped

1 tablespoon chili powder

½ teaspoon ground cumin

⅛ teaspoon cayenne

½ teaspoon salt

Topping:

¾ cup unbleached flour

¾ cup yellow cornmeal

1½ teaspoons salt

3 teaspoons baking powder

2 teaspoons sugar

¾ cup nonfat milk

1 egg

2 tablespoons light olive oil

- Bring the beans and the ¾ teaspoon salt to a boil in enough water to cover by several inches. Reduce the heat and cook gently, uncovered, until tender (50 to 60 minutes). If necessary, add more water to the beans to keep them covered. Drain and set aside.

- While the beans are cooking, sauté the onion and green bell pepper in the olive oil until soft. Add the garlic, briefly stirring. Add the tomatoes, chili powder, cumin, cayenne, and salt. Cook, uncovered, until reduced to 2 cups, 30 to 40 minutes.

- Add the cooked beans and heat through.

- Lightly grease an 8-inch-square, stainless steel pan about 2 inches deep.

- Combine the flour, cornmeal, salt, baking powder, and sugar in a bowl.

- In another bowl, whisk together the milk, egg, and 2 tablespoons olive oil. Add to the flour mixture and stir just to combine.

- Spread the heated beans evenly in the greased 8-inch pan. Top evenly with the cornmeal mixture. Bake in a preheated 425°F oven until brown, 16 to 18 minutes.

6 servings

161

Corn-Topped Asparagus

If the available asparagus is too virile, peel the lower halves. The flavor and aroma of fresh asparagus deliciously complement the taste of the slightly browned corn topping.

1 pound asparagus, tough lower stems broken off

1 tablespoon plus 1 teaspoon (4 teaspoons) reduced-sodium soy sauce

2 teaspoons fresh ginger, grated fine

1 large garlic clove, minced

2 teaspoons toasted sesame seeds

¾ cup unbleached flour

¾ cup cornmeal

½ teaspoon salt

3 teaspoons baking powder

2 teaspoons sugar

1 egg, beaten

¾ cup nonfat milk

3 teaspoons sesame oil

2 teaspoons light olive oil

½ teaspoon light olive oil

- Lightly grease an 8-inch-square pan.
- Cut the asparagus diagonally into 1-inch-thick pieces.
- Combine the soy, ginger, and garlic in a small bowl.
- Toast the sesame seeds in a small pan until just turning golden brown and set aside.
- Combine the flour, cornmeal, salt, baking powder, and sugar in a bowl and set aside.
- Whisk together the egg, milk, sesame oil, and 2 teaspoons olive oil and set aside.
- Heat the ½ teaspoon olive oil in a large skillet over medium heat. Add the asparagus and the soy mixture and sauté for 1 minute. Stir in the sesame seeds and turn the mixture into the baking pan.
- Combine the flour mixture with the egg mixture and spread evenly and smoothly over the top of the asparagus.
- Bake at 425°F for 15 to 18 minutes until the top is golden.

6 servings

Curried Cauliflower

The cauliflower should be divided into small flowerets. Chunks will take too long to cook. This combination provides enough verve to make cauliflower fascinating.

8 ounces onion, sliced

1 teaspoon olive oil

3 large garlic cloves, minced

2 teaspoons turmeric

2 teaspoons ground coriander

1 tablespoon ground cumin

2 teaspoons garam masala

¼ teaspoon crushed red pepper flakes

salt

2½ pounds tomatoes, peeled and chopped

1¾ pounds cauliflower flowerets

rice

cilantro, chopped

- Sauté the onion in the olive oil until brown, about 20 minutes. Remove the pan from the heat to cool briefly.
- Add the garlic, turmeric, coriander, cumin, garam masala, pepper flakes, and salt to the pan and stir.
- Add the tomatoes and cook until they are pulpy and thick, 25 to 30 minutes.
- Add the cauliflower, cover, and simmer until tender, 6 to 8 minutes.
- Serve over hot, cooked rice and garnish with cilantro.

4 to 6 servings

Curried Eggplant With Potatoes and Tomatoes

Eggplant, or *brinjal,* is a favorite ingredient in many Indian dishes. Combining it with potatoes and tomatoes makes this a satisfying main dish. In India, potatoes are often combined with rice or high-carbohydrate foods. They are considered vegetables, and they can absorb the aromatic and intense spices the Indians so love.

1 small onion (roughly 8 ounces), chopped

1 teaspoon olive oil

3 large garlic cloves, minced

2 teaspoons turmeric

2 tablespoons ground coriander

3 teaspoons ground cumin

¼ teaspoon cayenne, optional

3 pounds tomatoes, peeled and cut into 1-inch cubes

1 pound eggplant, cut into ½-inch cubes

1 tablespoon fresh ginger, grated fine

2½ pounds russet potatoes, peeled and cut into 1-inch cubes

salt

rice

cilantro, chopped, for garnish

- Sauté the onion in the olive oil until tender. Add the garlic, briefly stirring.
- Add the turmeric, coriander, cumin, and cayenne. Sauté 1 to 2 minutes.
- Add the tomatoes, eggplant, and ginger. Simmer, covered, for 20 minutes.
- Add the potatoes to the pot. Continue cooking gently, covered, until the potatoes are tender, 20 to 25 minutes.
- Add salt.
- Serve with cooked rice and garnish with cilantro.

4 to 6 servings

Garbanzo Bean and Pea Curry

In India, cinnamon is considered a hot spice and is not used to flavor sweets. Cardamom is often used in its place in sweets. In this recipe, the cinnamon enhances the flavor of the other spices. The rather unusual combination of peas and garbanzo beans makes this a textural delight.

12 ounces onion, chopped

1 tablespoon fresh ginger, grated fine

1 tablespoon garlic, chopped

1 teaspoon olive oil

1 tablespoon curry powder

¼ teaspoon cinnamon

1½ teaspoons turmeric

¼ teaspoon coriander

¼ teaspoon cumin

1¾ pounds tomatoes, peeled and chopped

1 16-ounce can garbanzo beans, drained and rinsed

1 cup fresh peas, cooked

salt

pepper

rice

cilantro, chopped

Chutney (page 219)

plain, nonfat yogurt

- Purée the onion, ginger, garlic, and olive oil until very smooth. Cook for 6 minutes, stirring often.
- Add the curry powder, cinnamon, turmeric, coriander, and cumin. Stir to blend.
- Add the tomatoes and cook until they are thick and pulpy, about 20 minutes.
- Add the garbanzo beans and cooked peas. Continue cooking for 10 minutes.
- Add salt and pepper.
- Serve the curry over cooked rice and garnish with chopped cilantro.
- Chutney and plain, nonfat yogurt may be served on the side.

4 servings

Lentil Curry

This is a rich-tasting, spicy dish. Tomatoes, currants, apples, and bananas give this a light, fruity taste. Serve it with a spinach raita and chapatis.

1 teaspoon olive oil

12 ounces onion, chopped

4 large garlic cloves, minced

3 pounds tomatoes, peeled and chopped

¼ teaspoon turmeric

½ teaspoon cumin seeds, toasted and ground

1 tablespoon coriander seeds, toasted and ground

1 tablespoon fresh ginger, grated fine

¼ teaspoon cayenne, or ½ small red chili pepper

1 cup lentils, sorted and rinsed

½ teaspoon salt

4½ cups water

½ cup currants

1 green banana, peeled and cut into thin slices

white rice or basmati rice

Chutney (page 219)

cilantro

- In a sauce pan, heat the olive oil over medium heat. Add the onion and sauté until onion is brown, about 20 to 25 minutes. Remove the pan from heat for a short while before adding the garlic and sautéing, briefly stirring.

- Add the tomatoes, turmeric, cumin, coriander, ginger, and cayenne. Bring to a boil, reduce heat, and simmer, uncovered, until soft and pulpy, 15 to 20 minutes.

- While the tomatoes are cooking, combine the lentils, salt, and water in a pan, bring to a boil, reduce heat, and boil gently until tender, 20 to 25 minutes. Drain.

- Combine the lentils and tomatoes.

- Add the currants and simmer for 10 minutes. Add the sliced banana and cook 5 minutes.

- Serve with cooked rice, chutney, and chopped cilantro leaves.

6 servings

Tomato-Potato Curry

The potatoes in this curry can be cooked in the Indian fashion, until quite soft. Perhaps a few could be mashed with the back of a spoon, especially if the tomatoes are too juicy. The spice blend yields a distinctive flavor.

8 ounces onion, chopped

1 teaspoon olive oil

3 tablespoons ginger, chopped

3 large garlic cloves, minced; about 1 tablespoon

3 pounds tomatoes, peeled and chopped

5 cardamom pods, crushed to release tiny black seeds, which should then be crushed

1½ teaspoons turmeric

1½ teaspoons garam masala

⅛ teaspoon cayenne

1¼ pounds peeled russet potatoes, cut into 1-inch cubes

salt

rice

Chutney (page 219)

cilantro, chopped, for garnish

- Sauté the onion in the olive oil until tender. Add the ginger and garlic and sauté for 1 minute.
- Add the tomatoes, cardamom, turmeric, garam masala, and cayenne. Cook for 5 minutes.
- Add the potatoes and cook slowly, covered, until tender, 20 to 25 minutes, stirring occasionally.
- Add salt.
- Serve with cooked rice and chutney.
- Garnish with cilantro.

4 servings

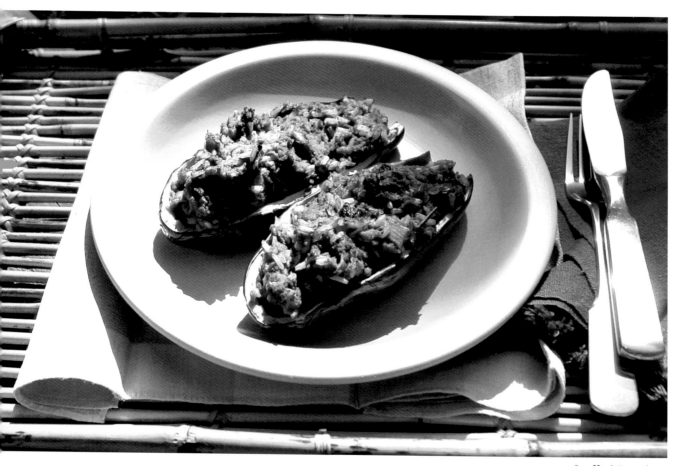

Stuffed Eggplant

Stuffed Eggplant

This is a small dish that can be multiplied by 2 or 4, if you like.

¼ cup brown rice, uncooked

1 eggplant, about 1 pound, or 2 eggplants, each ½ pound

8 ounces onion, chopped

1 teaspoon olive oil

3 large garlic cloves, minced

1½ teaspoons ground coriander

1½ teaspoons ground cumin

⅛ teaspoon cayenne

1 cup tomatoes, peeled and chopped

⅛ teaspoon cinnamon

¼ cup raisins

salt

Chutney (page 219)

- Cook the rice until just done, 25 minutes. Drain and set aside.
- Cut the stem from the eggplant and slice it in half lengthwise.
- Using a melon baller, carefully scoop out the flesh, leaving a ¼-inch-thick shell.
- Pulse the eggplant in a food processor to get a coarse consistency.
- Sauté the onion in the olive oil until tender. Add the garlic, briefly stirring.
- Add the spices, briefly stirring.
- Add the tomatoes and cook, uncovered, until soft and most of the liquid has evaporated (about 10 minutes).
- Add the eggplant to the tomatoes, cover, and cook gently until soft (about 3 minutes).
- Combine the rice, eggplant-tomato mixture, cinnamon, raisins, and salt.
- Divide the mixture evenly between the eggplant shells.
- Bake, covered, in a lightly greased baking dish at 350°F until hot and the shells are tender, about 45 minutes.
- Serve with chutney.

2 servings

169

Eggplant and Tomatoes on Brown Rice

Do use one of the more distinctive basils in this recipe, such as true Thai or African Blue.

1¼ pounds eggplant, cut into very small cubes

2 pounds tomatoes, peeled and chopped

3 large garlic cloves, minced

¼ cup fresh basil, chopped (or 1 teaspoon dry basil)

⅛ teaspoon crushed red pepper flakes

salt

4 teaspoons balsamic vinegar

brown rice

basil, chopped

- Combine the eggplant, tomatoes, garlic, basil, and pepper flakes in a pot. Simmer until tender, 25 to 30 minutes.
- While the vegetables simmer, start cooking the rice. This can be done by gently boiling the rice for about 25 minutes or more, until a small sample tastes as tender as you prefer.
- Add salt.
- Stir in the vinegar.
- Serve with brown rice and garnish with basil.

4 servings

Lentils With Browned Onion

These lentils, and the following baked version, depend on the caramel-like taste of really brown—but not burned—onions.

10 ounces brown lentils, sorted and
    rinsed
1 pound onion, chopped
1 teaspoon olive oil
1½ teaspoons salt
pepper
brown rice

- In a pot, add water to cover the lentils by 2 inches. Simmer rapidly until tender, about 25 to 30 minutes. Add salt during the last 5 minutes.
- While the lentils are cooking, sauté the onion in the olive oil until very brown, about 20 minutes or more.
- When the lentils are done, drain them and add additional salt, if necessary, and the pepper.
- Stir in the browned onion and serve with brown rice cooked as in the preceding recipe.

4 servings

Lentils Baked With Rice

The browned onion, together with the cumin seed, gives the lentils enough flavor support to make this baked dish quite flavorful.

1 onion (about 8 ounces), chopped

1 teaspoon olive oil

1½ cups lentils, sorted and rinsed

1 teaspoon salt

¾ teaspoon cumin seed, toasted and ground

1 cup rice, uncooked

1¾ cups Vegetable Broth (page 58), heated

¾ teaspoon salt

pepper

plain, nonfat yogurt

Chutney (page 219)

- Sauté the onion in the olive oil until very brown, 20 to 25 minutes.
- Cook the lentils in water to cover with the ½ teaspoon salt, until done, 20 to 30 minutes. Drain.
- In a heavy casserole, combine the browned onion, cooked lentils, cumin, rice, heated broth, ½ teaspoon salt, and pepper. Bring to a simmer.
- Bake, tightly covered, at 400°F for 25 minutes.
- Fluff with a fork and serve with yogurt and chutney.

4 to 6 servings

Spicy Lentils With Couscous

The spice results from the addition of cumin, turmeric, and pepper.

Lentils:

1 teaspoon olive oil

1 onion (about 8 ounces), chopped

4 large garlic cloves, minced

2 tablespoons fresh ginger, grated fine

8 ounces lentils, sorted and rinsed

5½ cups Vegetable Broth (page 58)

2 teaspoons cumin seed, toasted and
    ground

1½ teaspoons turmeric

¼ teaspoon crushed red pepper flakes

salt

Couscous:

2 cups Vegetable Broth (page 58)

1⅓ cups couscous

Lentils:

- In a saucepan, heat the olive oil and sauté the onion until soft.
- Add the garlic and ginger to the pan and sauté briefly.
- Add the lentils, vegetable broth, ground cumin seed, turmeric, and pepper flakes. Bring to a boil, reduce heat, and simmer, partially covered, for 40 to 45 minutes or until the lentils are tender.
- Add salt and serve with couscous.

Couscous:

- Bring the vegetable broth to a boil.
- Stir in the couscous, remove from heat, and cover.
- Let stand for 5 minutes and fluff with a fork.

6 servings

Lima Beans

Also known as butter beans, these beans were discovered in Lima, Peru. If you happen upon the fresh beans in a farmer's market, try them. They have an entirely different—and better—flavor than those you purchase in the store.

1 pound large, dried lima beans, sorted and rinsed

12 cups water

1 onion (about 8 ounces), chopped

1½ teaspoons salt

2 teaspoons Angostura Worcestershire sauce

1½ teaspoons white wine vinegar

1½ teaspoons dry mustard

1 tablespoon plus 1 teaspoon dark molasses

1 tablespoon plus 1 teaspoon chili sauce

¾ cup bean liquid

pepper

- Simmer the beans in the water with the onion and salt until just done, 1 to 1¼ hours. Be careful not to overcook the beans. Drain, reserving ¾ cup bean liquid, and rinse gently with cold water.

- Combine Worcestershire, vinegar, mustard, molasses, chili sauce, and bean liquid in a double boiler. Add the drained beans and pepper.

- Heat through.

6 servings

Red Bell Peppers Stuffed With Curried Rice

Stuffed peppers, especially red bell peppers, look appetizing as they are served steaming-hot from the oven.

2 large red bell peppers, washed, halved lengthwise, including the stems, and seeded

¾ cup rice

1 teaspoon olive oil

2 teaspoons curry powder

½ cup raisins

¼ cup scallions, sliced

¾ teaspoon salt

¾ cup water

Chutney (page 219)

- Plunge the pepper halves into boiling water for 2 minutes, drain, and set aside.
- Boil the rice for 12 minutes and drain. Transfer to a bowl.
- Heat the olive oil in a small pan. Add the curry powder and cook for 1 to 2 minutes, stirring.
- Add the raisins, scallions, salt, and water. Cook gently for 4 minutes and combine with the rice.
- Fill the pepper halves equally with the rice mixture and bake, covered, at 350°F until hot, 40 to 45 minutes.
- Serve with chutney.

4 servings

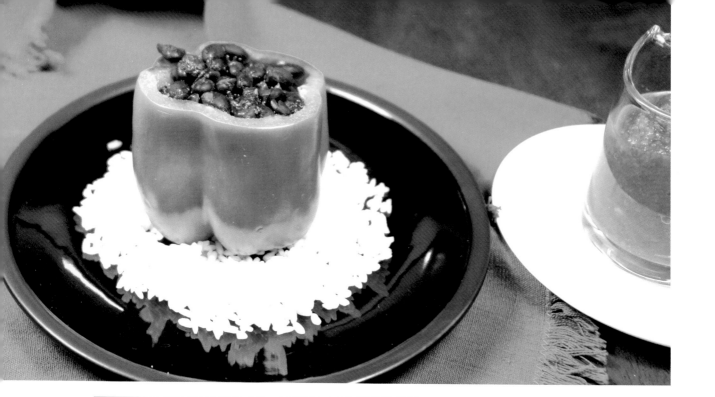

Orange Peppers Stuffed With Black Beans With Orange Pepper Sauce

A Halloween dish with stunning orange colors. This is not a tower dish floating on a slippery substrate that challenges the diner, with knife in hand, to cut a portion to eat without having the pepper reappear on her lap or on the floor.

Beans:

8 ounces black beans, sorted and rinsed

8 ounces onion, chopped

2 large garlic cloves, minced

1 bay leaf

¾ teaspoon dry oregano

¼ teaspoon crushed red pepper flakes

¼ cup parsley, chopped

1½ cups Vegetable Broth (page 58)

3½ cups water

1½ teaspoons salt

Beans:

- Combine the black beans, onion, garlic, bay leaf, oregano, pepper flakes, parsley, broth, water, and salt in a pot. Bring to a boil, reduce heat, and simmer, uncovered, until beans are tender and the sauce is thick, 1¾ to 2 hours. Add additional water, if necessary, to keep the beans just covered. Set aside.

(continued)

176

Sauce:

1 onion (about 8 ounces), chopped

1 teaspoon olive oil

2 large garlic cloves, minced

1 pound 4 ounces orange bell peppers, seeded and chopped

1 14-ounce can crushed tomatoes in thick purée

$1/8$ teaspoon crushed red pepper flakes

salt

To Assemble:

4 orange bell peppers that stand up, tops sliced off and seeded

1 cup rice, uncooked

Sauce:

- Sauté the onion in the olive oil until soft. Add the garlic, briefly stirring.
- Add the chopped bell peppers, tomatoes, and pepper flakes. Simmer, covered, for 20 minutes or until the peppers are soft.
- Purée and add salt. Set aside.

To Assemble:

- Drop the 4 peppers into boiling water for 2 minutes. Drain and rinse with cold water. Let stand until cool enough to handle.
- Divide the black beans equally among the 4 peppers.
- Place in baking dish and cover.
- Bake at 350°F until hot, 30 to 40 minutes.
- While the peppers are heating, boil the rice and drain. Set aside and keep warm.
- To serve, divide the rice equally among the 4 plates. Place 1 pepper on each plate on top of the rice.
- Serve with the heated pepper sauce.

4 servings

177

Polenta With Red Bell Pepper Sauce

Polenta, Italian cornmeal, develops an intense corn taste when cooked slowly. It will stick to the pan bottom if it is not stirred or whisked almost constantly. The pepper sauce adds the right intense flavor to contrast with the relative blandness of the polenta.

Polenta:

1½ cups polenta

6 cups Vegetable Broth (page 58), cool or at room temperature

1½ teaspoons salt

Sauce:

1 pound onion, chopped

1 teaspoon olive oil, divided

2 garlic cloves, minced

1½ pounds tomatoes, peeled and chopped

1 pound red bell pepper, seeded and chopped

8 ounces green bell pepper, seeded and chopped

salt

pepper

¼ cup cilantro, chopped

- Combine the polenta, broth, and salt in a pan. Bring to a boil while whisking constantly. Reduce heat and continue whisking for 20 minutes. Pour immediately into an 8-by 12-inch flat baking dish. Let cool at room temperature and chill.

- Sauté the onion in the olive oil until tender. Add the garlic, briefly stirring.

- Add the tomatoes to the pot and cook for 10 minutes, uncovered. Add the bell peppers and continue cooking, uncovered, for 25 minutes or until the liquid has evaporated. Purée and return to a clean pan. Add salt and pepper.

- Cut the polenta into 18 squares. Heat ½ teaspoon olive oil in each of 2 nonstick skillets and add the polenta squares. Cook for 30 minutes, turning only once.

- Heat the sauce and stir in the cilantro. Divide the sauce among the polenta squares.

6 servings

Polenta With Vegetables: Bell Peppers, Zucchini, and Cauliflower

Adding zucchini and cauliflower to the sauce makes this a more substantial dish while retaining the contrast between the vegetables and the polenta.

Sauce:

4 pounds tomatoes, peeled and chopped

1 tablespoon garlic

1 teaspoon olive oil

8 ounces onion, chopped

1 pound assorted bell peppers, seeded and cut into small strips

4 ounces cauliflower, cut into small pieces

2 small zucchini, cut into small pieces

salt

pepper

Sauce:

- Cook the tomatoes in a large pan until they are soft and pulpy, about 30 minutes.

- Sauté the garlic in the olive oil briefly, add the onion, and sauté until soft. Add the bell peppers, cauliflower, and zucchini and cook until crisp-tender.

- Add the vegetable mixture to the tomatoes and cook gently for about 10 minutes.

- Add salt and pepper.

Polenta:

1½ cups polenta

6 cups Vegetable Broth (page 58)

Polenta:

- Combine the polenta and room-temperature broth. Add salt.

- Cook over medium heat for about 25 minutes until thickened. The mixture should still be creamy.

- Divide the polenta among 6 serving dishes and top it with the sauce.

6 servings

179

Rice and Beans With Ginger and Soy

Soy sauce gives the beans a savory flavor.

1 cup dried pink beans, sorted and
  rinsed
1½ teaspoons salt
1 cup rice, uncooked
1 teaspoon olive oil
1½ cups scallions, sliced
2½ teaspoons fresh ginger, grated fine
½ teaspoon salt
4 tablespoons low-sodium soy sauce
cilantro, chopped, for garnish

- Add enough water to the beans to cover by 2 inches. Add the 1½ teaspoons salt and simmer, uncovered, until the beans are tender, about 1¼ hours. Drain and keep warm.

- Cook the rice, uncovered, in water to cover for 12 minutes. Drain and keep warm.

- Heat the olive oil in a heavy pan and stir-fry the scallions and ginger for 1 minute.

- Add the beans and stir well. Then add the ½ teaspoon salt and the soy sauce. Cover and simmer for 2 minutes.

- Add the rice to the beans and stir well.

- Garnish with the cilantro.

4 to 6 servings

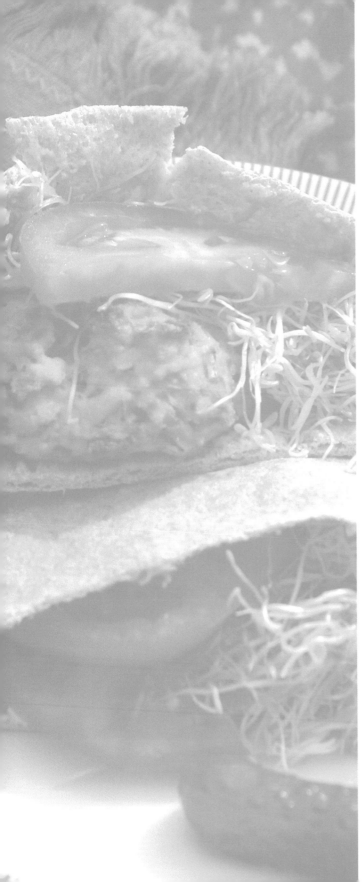

Tofu and Tempeh

Tofu is a great, healthful food that should not inspire foreboding in the diner. That white slab of wonderfully changed soybeans is a significant source of protein, and if the brand is carefully chosen, it is low in fat. The problem is that tofu doesn't look like a beautifully browned hunk of steak. Cut into slabs, tofu can be browned and decorated with bits of attractive vegetables—and napped with a colorful and deeply flavored sauce. But! Once you cut into the slab, you reveal the soft underbelly of tofu—and a white interior that looks rather like the tofu before you started.

The solution, I believe, is to cut the tofu into small, *thin* pieces that can be sautéed until brown and dense and then coated with a spicy sauce. Marinating tofu does help add some flavor to smaller cuts. Of course, it also can be disguised entirely by incorporating it in mayonnaise or by crumbling the tofu and forming it into burger shapes that can be browned beautifully. Very thin-sliced tofu can also be cooked slowly while brushing the pieces with a flavored liquid as simple as very low-sodium soy sauce, giving the end product a crisp, wafer-like appearance.

(continued)

181

Another soybean food, tempeh (or tempe), is fermented soy. Tempeh is about 40 percent protein, and like tofu, is a rich source of lysine, an amino acid in which rice is deficient. Fermentation makes the lysine available to human digestion. Tempeh probably originated in Indonesia and is a staple of the diet throughout Southeast Asia. Tempeh is firmer in texture than tofu, and when sliced thin, it lends itself to marination. Its dense chewiness is certainly appealing.

The importance of both of these soy-based foods will, no doubt, become more and more significant throughout Asia, India, and Africa, where chicken forms a major source of protein. Destruction of poultry stocks in these countries in the attempt to control the spread of the deadly H5N1 avian flu virus may result in widespread nutritional deficiencies except in those places where soy-based foods are consumed daily and have been for centuries.

Tempeh—Marinated

Tempeh acquires a nutty flavor when browned, as in this dish. It is usually unsalted, unlike soy sauce, so the added soy sauce does not make the marinated end-product too salty. Tempeh makes an excellent sandwich filling. Try it with crunchy sprouted whole-wheat bread topped with juicy tomato slices and some sharp-tasting grainy mustard. For a smoky, hot flavor, use ground chipotle chili instead of crushed red bell pepper.

¼ cup low-sodium soy sauce

1½ tablespoons rice vinegar

3 garlic cloves, minced

1 tablespoon fresh ginger, grated fine

⅛ teaspoon crushed red bell pepper

4 ounces soy tempeh, sliced into ¼-inch pieces

½ teaspoon olive oil

- Combine the soy sauce, vinegar, garlic, ginger, and crushed pepper in a small pan. Bring to a boil briefly. Add the tempeh and remove from heat.

- Let marinate at room temperature for 2 hours, covered.

- Remove the tempeh pieces from the marinade. Sauté the tempeh in ½ teaspoon olive oil in a nonstick skillet over medium heat for 20 to 30 minutes until nicely browned.

- Serve with cooked apples, applesauce, or pineapple salsa.

2 servings

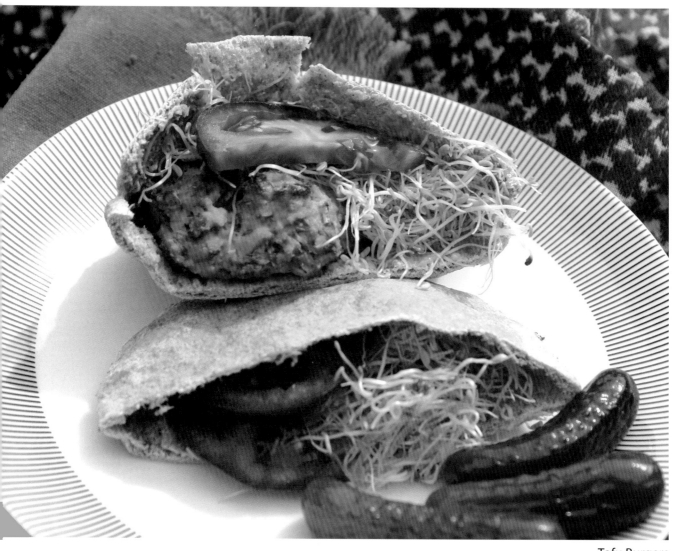

Tofu Burgers

Tofu Burgers

These burgers will survive, flavor intact, after freezing either before or after baking. To make the process easier, chill the ingredients before forming into burgers. If you will use these in a sandwich or pita bread half, make them flat.

2 pounds extra-firm tofu

8 ounces onion, chopped

1 large carrot, grated

1½ cups celery, chopped

1 teaspoon olive oil

2 teaspoons dried basil

1 cup fresh whole-wheat bread crumbs

⅓ cup parsley, minced

2 tablespoons Dijon mustard

5 tablespoons low-sodium soy sauce

3 egg whites, lightly beaten

pepper

- Rinse the tofu and slice each cake into about 12 pieces. Drain on several thicknesses of paper towels for 30 minutes.

- Place the tofu slices into a clean tea towel. Twist the tea towel to seal the tofu inside. Knead and squeeze the tofu vigorously in order to remove as much water as possible. The tofu should look dry and crumbly.

- While the tofu is draining, sauté the onion, carrot, and celery in the olive oil until tender.

- Combine the vegetables and tofu with the remaining ingredients.

- Shape into 8 burgers, each a generous ¼ cup. Use an ice cream scoop, if you have one, to measure the portions.

- Bake on a lightly greased pan at 375°F for 30 minutes, until lightly browned.

- Serve on your favorite fat-free bread, toasted, with condiments such as lettuce, tomato, sprouts, pickles, catsup, mustard, and onion.

8 servings

Mushroom Gravy

A flavorful accompaniment for tofu burgers, this gravy freezes well.

$\frac{1}{3}$ cup plus 1 tablespoon unbleached
  flour
2 cups Vegetable Broth (page 58)
8 ounces onion, minced
4 ounces mushrooms, minced
1 teaspoon garlic, minced
1 cup dry, red wine
1 tablespoon low-sodium soy sauce
salt
pepper

- Put the flour into a heavy 8-inch skillet. Cook over medium-high heat, stirring constantly, until light brown, about 10 minutes. Turn the heat down, if necessary, to avoid burning. Sift the flour into a bowl and set aside.
- Combine the vegetable broth, onion, mushrooms, and garlic in a saucepan. Bring to a boil, reduce heat, and simmer for 15 minutes.
- Stir in the wine and soy sauce.
- Gradually whisk in the browned flour.
- Continue to simmer, stirring occasionally, until thickened, about 45 minutes.
- Add salt and pepper.

3 cups

Marinated Tofu

Marinating the tofu and baking it in the marinade results in a more flavorful and chewy filet of tofu. Try frozen, thawed tofu for this dish. Freezing opens lacunae in the tofu to accept the marinade.

¾ cup dry, red wine

½ cup low-sodium soy sauce

¼ cup garlic-flavored red wine vinegar

1 cup water

3 large garlic cloves, sliced

5 whole cloves

Use a generous stem with leaves attached for the following herbs, if you can:

  2 teaspoons dried oregano

  2 teaspoons dried marjoram

  1 teaspoon dried thyme

pepper

1 pound firm tofu, rinsed and sliced into ½-inch pieces, dried on paper towels for 20 to 30 minutes

- Combine wine, soy sauce, vinegar, water, garlic, cloves, oregano, marjoram, thyme, and pepper in a small pan.
- Simmer for 10 minutes.
- Arrange the dried tofu slices in a shallow dish in a single layer. Pour the marinade over the tofu slices.
- Cover and refrigerate for 3 to 4 days, turning several times.
- Lightly oil 1 or 2 nonstick skillets, big enough to hold the tofu slices in 1 layer. Using care to avoid breaking the tofu slices, add them to the heated skillets. Cook over medium heat until the slices are brown. Turn the slices carefully and repeat the process until well-browned.
- Arrange the slices in close order in a shallow baking dish. Add the marinade and bake at 350°F until quite firm, about 1 hour.
- Serve with cooked apples or applesauce.

4 servings

187

Tofu With Soy and Turmeric

This dish is superb. Its success depends on slow cooking over moderate to low heat. It is absolutely necessary to repeatedly turn the tofu slices over, brushing them lightly, then doing so again and again—as many as 10 times. If the slices are thin, the end result will be a crisp wafer of tofu, delightfully crumbly and intensely flavored. The resulting wafers will make an outstanding tofu, lettuce, and tomato sandwich. Or serve them with pancakes in the morning. Use low-fat tofu, if you can; it will be more fragile but will yield a more consistently crisp wafer. Don't be afraid to move the tofu with your fingers while it is crisping in the skillet. These wafers do not reheat well; they become tough and leathery. Make only enough to eat at once.

1 teaspoon turmeric

1/3 cup low-sodium soy sauce

1 1-pound package of extra-firm tofu, rinsed and sliced into 12 to 13 pieces and dried on paper towels for 20 minutes

- Combine the turmeric and soy.

- Arrange the tofu slices in a single layer in 2 nonstick skillets. Brush each slice with the turmeric-soy mixture. Turn the slices and brush again. Turn the heat on low and cook until the tofu is crisp, 45 to 60 minutes. Continue brushing and turning while the tofu cooks, using all the sauce.

- Serve with cooked apples, applesauce, or Pineapple Salsa (page 224).

2 to 3 servings

Spicy Ginger Tofu

The peppery flavor of this tofu dish will distract you from the fact that you are eating tofu!

1 pound extra-firm tofu
½ bunch cilantro, chopped
¼ cup lemon juice
2 teaspoons crushed red pepper flakes
10 large garlic cloves, sliced
1¼ cups Vegetable Broth (page 58)
¼ cup ginger, chopped fine
½ to 1 teaspoon olive oil

- Rinse the tofu and cut crosswise into 13 to 14 slices. Drain on paper towels for 30 minutes.
- Combine the cilantro, lemon juice, red pepper flakes, garlic, broth, and ginger in a flat 15- by 10- by 2-inch dish. Carefully add the tofu slices to the marinade and coat all sides. Cover and let stand at room temperature for 4 hours. Turn the tofu slices several times.
- Coat 2 nonstick skillets lightly with olive oil and heat. Add the tofu slices and cook over low heat for 45 minutes, until the tofu is browned and firm, turning frequently.
- Serve with Pineapple Salsa (page 224).

2 to 3 servings

Tortilla Bean Casserole

What is a casserole? It is certainly a dish, usually ceramic or glass, often containing—as this casserole does—a mixture of compatible ingredients, frequently layered. It is not a *tian*, which is a shallow dish topped with cheese. This casserole is rich with tomatoes and spices. The tortillas should retain their integrity, giving a textural contrast that pleases.

Beans:

8 ounces onion, chopped

1 teaspoon olive oil

6 ounces pinto beans, sorted and rinsed

¾ teaspoon salt

water

4 corn tortillas, cut into eighths

cilantro

tomatillo salsa—Apple-Tomatillo Salsa (page 223) or a good prepared salsa

Sauce:

12 ounces onion, chopped

1 teaspoon olive oil

3 large garlic cloves, minced

5 pounds tomatoes, peeled and chopped

3 teaspoons ground cumin

3 tablespoons fresh oregano, chopped

2 teaspoons seeded jalapeño, minced

1½ cups green bell pepper, seeded and chopped

salt

Beans:

- Sauté the onion in the olive oil until soft.
- Add the beans and the salt to the pot. Add enough water to cover the beans by 4 inches. Bring to a boil, reduce the heat, and simmer for 1 to 1¼ hours or until done.

(continued)

Sauce:

- Sauté the onion in the olive oil until soft.
- Add the garlic, briefly stirring.
- Add the tomatoes, cumin, oregano, and jalapeño to the pot. Simmer the sauce, uncovered, until it is no longer wet, 1½ to 2 hours.
- Add the green bell pepper and simmer 5 minutes longer.
- Add salt and stir in the drained beans.

Tortillas:

- Bake the corn tortillas on a baking sheet at 400°F for 12 to 14 minutes until crisp.

To Assemble:

- Assemble the casserole in an 8- by 12-inch flat baking dish. Put a layer of sauce on the bottom, add a layer of tortillas, a layer of sauce, a layer of tortillas, and end with a layer of sauce.
- Bake the casserole, uncovered, in a 350°F oven for 30 minutes or until hot.
- Garnish with cilantro leaves and serve with tomatillo salsa.

6 servings

Tostadas With Tofu and Chayote

Chayote is another American native, a squash-like vegetable with a fine texture, resembling a green apple with a pear in its ancestry.

Tofu:

1 pound firm or extra-firm tofu, rinsed

3 tablespoons fresh lime juice

¼ cup plus 2 tablespoons tequila

2 teaspoons chili powder

1¼ teaspoons ground cumin

1½ teaspoons turmeric

¾ teaspoons salt

4 corn tortillas

cilantro, chopped

tomatillo salsa

plain, nonfat yogurt

Vegetables:

8 ounces onion, chopped

1 teaspoon olive oil

3 large garlic cloves, minced

1¼ pounds tomatoes, peeled and chopped

2½ teaspoons chili powder

1½ teaspoons ground cumin

⅛ teaspoon cayenne

1¼ pounds chayote, peeled and cut into ½-inch cubes

1 cup frozen baby lima beans, cooked

1½ cups red bell pepper, seeded and chopped

salt

Tofu:

- Cut the tofu into thin slices, about 16 or more. Dry the slices on paper towels for 30 minutes.
- Combine the lime juice, tequila, chili powder, cumin, turmeric, and salt.
- Carefully arrange the tofu slices in a single layer in 2 large nonstick skillets.
- Brush each slice with the lime-tequila mixture. Carefully turn the slices over. Turn the heat to low and brush the slices again. Continue brushing and turning the slices until the lime-tequila mixture is gone. Continue cooking and turning until the slices are crisp, about 45 to 60 minutes.

(continued)

Vegetables:

- Sauté the onion in the olive oil until soft. Add the garlic, briefly stirring.
- Add the tomatoes, chili powder, cumin, and cayenne. Cook, uncovered, until the tomatoes are thick and pulpy, about 20 minutes.
- Add the chayote, cover, and simmer 25 to 30 minutes or until tender.
- Add the cooked lima beans and red bell pepper. Continue cooking, covered, over low heat for 5 minutes.
- Add salt.

Tortillas:

- Bake the tortillas on a cookie sheet at 400°F for 10 minutes or until crisp, turning several times.
- Serve the hot tortillas topped with the chayote mixture.
- Divide the tofu slices equally among the 4 tortillas.
- Garnish with the cilantro.
- Serve with tomatillo salsa and plain, nonfat yogurt.

4 servings

Vegetable Casserole

This vegetable mixture could be honored with the French title of *tian*, since it is cooked in a shallow dish and topped with well-browned bread crumbs. No matter what you call it, it is a robust dish combining vegetables, tomatoes, and beans in a nutritious and balanced way.

1 pound plus 2 ounces cauliflower flowerets

10 ounces green beans, ends removed and broken into 1-inch lengths; or 10 ounces zucchini, cut into ½-inch pieces

1 red bell pepper, seeded and cut into 1-inch pieces

1 green bell pepper, seeded and cut into 1-inch pieces

1 teaspoon olive oil

1 16-ounce can red kidney beans, drained and rinsed

1 28-ounce can crushed tomatoes in purée

6 tablespoons double-concentrated Italian tomato paste (comes in a tube)

1 teaspoon dried oregano

¾ teaspoon salt

pepper

1 cup fresh whole-wheat bread crumbs

- Steam the cauliflower until crisp-tender, 4 to 7 minutes. Set aside.
- Boil the green beans until just tender, 5 to 10 minutes, and drain. Set aside. If using zucchini, do not cook it.
- In a pan large enough to hold all the ingredients except the bread crumbs, sauté the bell peppers in the olive oil until crisp-tender.
- Add the remaining ingredients except the bread crumbs and bring to a boil. Stir gently several times.
- Turn into a 9- by 13-inch pan. Bake, uncovered, at 375°F until hot, 25 to 30 minutes.
- Sprinkle the bread crumbs evenly on top and broil until golden.

6 servings

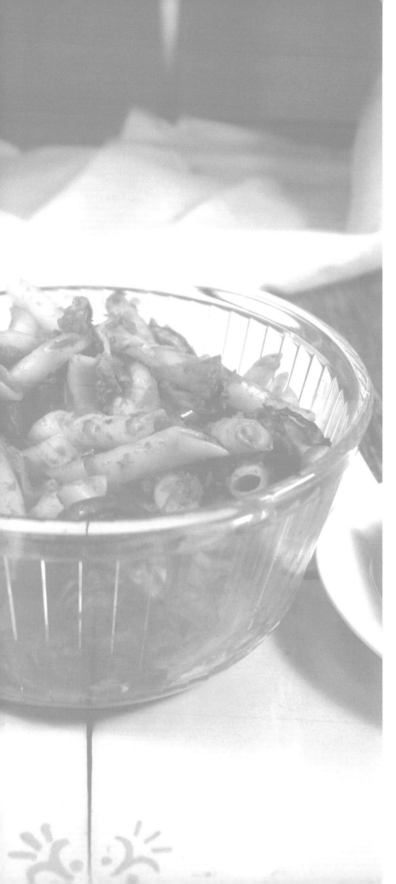

Pasta

The pasta in these recipes should be cooked al dente, that is, with some bite remaining. Start by using the package directions; you may find it useful to taste a strand. The weight of pasta to be prepared for one serving will vary with the eater, but *roughly* 2 ounces per person is a good departure point.

Broccoli-Tomato Gratin

This is an excellent, very low-fat dish. It could be compared to a delicious layered dish like lasagna.

16 ounces plain, nonfat cottage cheese

2 tablespoons grated Parmesan cheese

2 tablespoons sauce and gravy flour (pulverized flour)

2 egg whites

1 tablespoon plus 1 teaspoon fresh oregano, chopped

2 tablespoons fresh basil, chopped

1 tablespoon plus 1 teaspoon fresh thyme, chopped

pepper

1½ pounds broccoli (trimmed weight), cut into 6-inch lengths

2¾ cups tomato sauce, fresh, or commercial nonfat pasta sauce

- Purée the cottage cheese, Parmesan cheese, flour, egg whites, herbs, and pepper until just smooth. Do not over-purée.
- Steam the broccoli in 2 batches until crisp-tender, 3 to 5 minutes.
- Arrange half the broccoli in a 9-by 13-inch pan.
- Top with the cheese mixture.
- Arrange the remaining broccoli over the cheese mixture.
- Top with the tomato sauce.
- Bake, uncovered, at 375°F until heated through, 30 to 35 minutes.
- Serve with freshly cooked pasta.

4 to 6 servings

Broccoli and Cherry Tomatoes With Pasta

Fresh, organic broccoli can have an almost sweet flavor that accords well with the sweet-tart character of the cherry tomatoes.

2 cups broccoli, chopped

12 ounces cherry tomatoes, stems removed and washed

4 ounces onion, chopped

1 teaspoon olive oil

3 large garlic cloves, minced

¼ teaspoon crushed red pepper flakes

3 tablespoons fresh basil, chopped

½ teaspoon salt

4 ounces spaghetti, uncooked, broken into 2-inch lengths

- Steam the broccoli until crisp-tender and set aside.
- Halve the cherry tomatoes and set aside.
- Sauté the onion in the olive oil until tender. Add the garlic, briefly stirring.
- Add the tomatoes, pepper flakes, basil, and salt to the pot. Cook, covered, until hot (3 to 4 minutes).
- Add the broccoli and heat through (2 to 3 minutes).
- Cook the pasta, timing it to be done at the same time as the vegetables. Drain and mix with the vegetables.

2 large or 4 small servings

197

Brussels Sprouts and Pasta With Mustard Wine Sauce

Brussels sprouts can be too cabbagey in flavor. A wine sauce rich in grainy mustard flavor, added after the sprouts cook, can add a tangy coating. Be sure the sprouts are just done, still a bit crunchy. And, be sure you use fresh, small, mild sprouts. Absolutely avoid sprouts that have yellow or pale outer leaves or that are speckled with mold. If you buy large globes and remove the outer leaves, they will still be strongly flavored. Try a local farmer's market.

You may have to add more wine and more mustard if the sauce is over-reduced.

4 large garlic cloves, minced

1 teaspoon olive oil

4 tablespoons Dijon mustard

3 tablespoons lemon juice

1 cup dry, white wine

½ teaspoon caraway seeds

6 ounces linguini, uncooked, broken into 3-inch lengths

14 ounces Brussels sprouts, trimmed and quartered

salt

pepper

parsley, chopped, for garnish

- Sauté the garlic briefly in the olive oil. Add the Dijon mustard, lemon juice, white wine, and caraway seeds to the garlic. Simmer the sauce for 3 to 4 minutes.
- Start cooking the pasta to be al dente.
- While the pasta cooks, steam the Brussels sprouts until crisp-tender (6 to 10 minutes).
- When the pasta is done, drain it well and toss it with the heated sauce, adding salt and pepper. Stir in the Brussels sprouts. Turn off the heat and let the mixture stand for 10 minutes, covered.
- Heat gently and serve.
- Garnish with parsley.

4 servings

Cauliflower and Leek Pasta Sauce

Leeks, peppers, and tomatoes with the flavor of tarragon make this a savory combination. See method for cleaning leeks on page 81.

1¼ cups leeks, sliced, pale green and white parts only, washed well

1 cup red bell pepper, chopped

1 teaspoon olive oil

3 garlic cloves, minced

2 pounds tomatoes, peeled and chopped

2 tablespoons fresh tarragon, chopped

2 tablespoons double-concentrated Italian tomato paste (comes in a tube)

8 ounces cauliflower flowerets

salt

pepper

8 ounces linguini or other pasta

- Sauté the leeks and peppers in the olive oil until just tender.

- Add the garlic, briefly stirring.

- Add the tomatoes, tarragon, and tomato paste to the pot. Simmer, uncovered, until the sauce thickens, 20 to 25 minutes.

- Add the cauliflower and continue simmering the sauce, uncovered, until tender, about 10 minutes.

- Add salt and pepper and serve over freshly cooked pasta.

4 servings

Chickpea Pasta Sauce

This is a favorite dish because of its beautifully thickened, flavorful sauce. It can provide over 20 grams of protein per serving. Furthermore, it is very easy to assemble. Canned chickpeas vary greatly in flavor, so choose a brand you have already tasted, if possible.

1 onion (about 8 ounces), chopped

1 teaspoon olive oil

4 garlic cloves, minced

2 16-ounce cans low-salt chickpeas

2 pounds tomatoes, peeled and chopped coarse

1½ cups Vegetable Broth (page 58)

1 cup dry, red wine

1 loosely packed cup chopped basil

salt

pepper

8 ounces spaghetti

- Sauté the onion in the olive oil until soft. Add the garlic, briefly stirring.
- Drain and rinse 1 can of chickpeas. Purée this can of chickpeas and the tomatoes together until very smooth. Add to the pot.
- Drain and rinse the remaining can of chickpeas and add to the pot along with the broth. Cook, uncovered, for 30 minutes, add the red wine and basil, and cook for an additional 30 minutes.
- Add salt and pepper.
- Serve over freshly cooked pasta.

4 servings

Chinese Noodles

With dry-roasted peanuts, this dish contains about the same amount of fat as ½ tablespoon of olive oil: 7 grams. The flavored oils, together with the nuts, make this a rich-tasting dish with a bit of crunch.

8 ounces fresh Chinese noodles

3 tablespoons low-sodium soy sauce

½ teaspoon sesame oil

½ teaspoon sesame chili oil

⅓ cup cilantro, chopped

½ cup scallions, sliced thin

½ ounce salted, dry-roasted peanuts, chopped coarse

- Cook the noodles according to package directions and drain well.
- Return the noodles to the pot and dry well over low heat, shaking the pot.
- Add the remaining ingredients, toss lightly, and heat briefly.

2 servings

Eggplant-Tomato Sauce

Choose small or torpedo-shaped eggplant, for it is less likely to be enrobed in a tough, chewy peel. You might test the peel before embarking on this dish by piercing the skin with your fingernail or a blunt knife. If in doubt, peel.

1 teaspoon olive oil

3 large garlic cloves, minced

1 pound eggplant, cut into ¼-inch cubes

1½ pounds tomatoes, peeled and chopped

1 teaspoon dried oregano

1 teaspoon dried basil

1 bay leaf

12 ounces tomato paste

1½ cups dry, white wine

salt

pepper

12 ounces pasta, cooked

- Heat the olive oil over low heat. Add the garlic, briefly stirring.
- Add the eggplant, tomatoes, herbs, bay leaf, tomato paste, and wine. Combine the ingredients and simmer, covered, until the vegetables are tender (50 to 60 minutes).
- Add salt and pepper.
- Serve over cooked pasta.

7 cups sauce; 6 servings

Green Bean Tomato Sauce for Pasta

The characteristic flavor of fresh green beans paired with the slight acidity of fresh tomatoes blends to make this a delicious pasta combination.

1 tablespoon garlic, minced

1 teaspoon olive oil

3½ pounds tomatoes, peeled and chopped

1 tablespoon fresh thyme, chopped

12 ounces green beans, ends removed and broken into 2-inch lengths

salt

pepper

8 ounces pasta

- Sauté the garlic in the olive oil briefly.
- Add the tomatoes and thyme to the pan. Simmer, uncovered, until the tomatoes are soft and the sauce is thick, 35 to 45 minutes.
- Boil the green beans until tender, 5 to 10 minutes, and drain.
- Add the cooked green beans to the thickened sauce. Simmer for 10 minutes.
- Add salt and pepper.
- Serve over cooked pasta.

4 servings

Lentil-Tomato Pasta Sauce

Leaving the lentils whole for this pasta dish adds some textural variety.

1 pound onion, chopped

1 teaspoon olive oil

3 large garlic cloves, minced

6 ounces lentils, sorted and rinsed

3½ cups water

3 pounds tomatoes, peeled and chopped

½ cup dry, red wine

1 bay leaf

1 tablespoon fresh oregano, chopped

¼ cup fresh basil, chopped

3 tablespoons double-concentrated Italian tomato paste (comes in a tube)

salt

pepper

2 to 3 ounces spaghetti or other pasta per person, cooked

parsley, chopped, for garnish

- Sauté the onion in the olive oil until tender. Add the garlic, briefly stirring.
- Add the lentils and water to the pot. Bring to a boil, reduce heat, and simmer, covered, until done, 25 to 30 minutes.
- Add the tomatoes, wine, bay leaf, oregano, basil, and tomato paste to the pot. Simmer, uncovered, until the sauce thickens, 40 to 45 minutes. Add salt and pepper.
- Serve over freshly cooked pasta.
- Garnish with parsley.

6 servings

204

Mushrooms to Top Pasta Sauce

Meaty—pardon the expression—mushrooms such as portobellos cut into pieces that can be carried on a spoon to the mouth suit this topping. Don't cook the mushrooms to a state of dryness. Let some of the juices remain by cooking gently. If necessary, add a bit of dry, white wine, such as chardonnay.

1 garlic clove, minced

1 teaspoon olive oil

8 ounces mushrooms, sliced

$\frac{1}{8}$ teaspoon of each of these dried herbs: basil, thyme, oregano, and rosemary

$\frac{1}{4}$ teaspoon paprika

salt

pepper

- Sauté the garlic in the olive oil briefly.
- Add the mushrooms, herbs, and paprika.
- Sauté until the mushrooms are tender, 5 to 8 minutes.
- Add salt and pepper.
- Spoon the mushrooms evenly over 2 servings of pasta topped with your favorite tomato pasta sauce.

2 servings

Orzo Baked With Tomatoes, Basil, and Oregano

Orzo is the pasta that resembles rice and lends itself well to a baked pasta dish. It can be seized on a fork with the tomatoes, thus avoiding the contortions involved in wrapping a long, slippery noodle on a fork.

8 ounces onion, chopped

1 teaspoon olive oil

3 large garlic cloves, minced

1½ pounds tomatoes, peeled and chopped

8 ounces orzo, uncooked

2 tablespoons fresh basil, chopped

1 tablespoon fresh oregano, chopped

salt

pepper

- Sauté the onion in the olive oil until soft. Add the garlic, briefly stirring.
- Add the tomatoes and cook, uncovered, for 10 minutes or until soft.
- Cook the orzo al dente and drain. Rinse with cold water and drain well.
- Combine the orzo, tomatoes, herbs, salt, and pepper.
- Bake, covered, in a shallow baking dish at 350°F until heated through, about 30 minutes.

6 to 8 servings

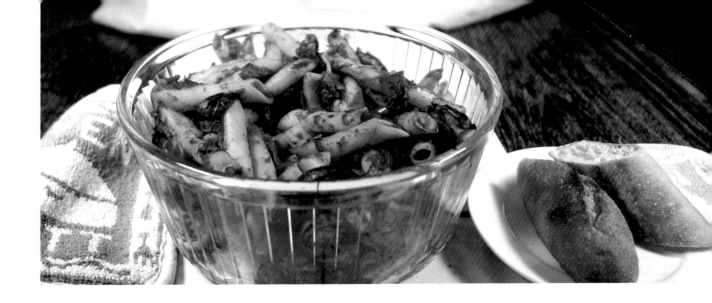

Penne Baked With Mushrooms and Eggplant

Penne is a good choice for a baked dish like this. The short corrugated or smooth tubes can be speared with panache—or even a fork.

1½ pounds small eggplants, not peeled, sliced ½-inch thick

1 teaspoon olive oil

10 ounces penne (less if the penne are large)

10 ounces mushrooms, sliced

4 large garlic cloves, minced

1 26-ounce jar of fat-free pasta sauce (Muir Glen is a good choice) or fresh homemade sauce

5 tablespoons double-concentrated Italian tomato paste (comes in a tube)

¾ cup dry, red wine

2 tablespoons fresh thyme, chopped

2 tablespoons fresh oregano, chopped

⅔ cup fresh basil, chopped

salt

pepper

- Brush the eggplant very lightly with olive oil and broil 4 inches from the flame for 4 to 5 minutes on each side.
- Cook the penne until barely tender. Drain and rinse the penne under cold water.
- Sauté the mushrooms in a skillet until tender and the liquid evaporates. Add the garlic briefly when the mushrooms are tender.
- Combine the pasta sauce, tomato paste, wine, mushrooms, eggplant, and herbs. Pour over the pasta, stir to combine, and add salt and pepper.
- Turn into a casserole and bake, uncovered, at 350°F until heated through, 30 to 40 minutes.

6 servings

207

Shells—Stuffed

Varying the shape of pasta adds greatly to the visual and textural appeal of pasta dishes.

16 giant pasta shells, uncooked

16 ounces plain, nonfat cottage cheese

¼ cup grated Asiago or Parmesan cheese

2 tablespoons sauce and gravy flour (pulverized flour)

2 egg whites

1 tablespoon plus 1 teaspoon fresh oregano, chopped

2 tablespoons fresh basil, chopped

1 tablespoon plus 1 teaspoon fresh thyme, chopped

1 teaspoon garlic, minced

pepper

2 cups fresh tomato sauce with sundried tomatoes or other fat-free pasta sauce

- Cook the shells al dente and rinse with cold water. Set aside.
- Purée the cottage cheese, Asiago or Parmesan, flour, egg whites, herbs, garlic, and pepper.
- Stuff the shells equally with the cheese mixture.
- Cover the bottom of a shallow baking dish, large enough to hold the shells, with a thin layer of sauce.
- Place the stuffed shells into the baking dish and top evenly with the remaining sauce.
- Cover and bake at 350°F until hot, 30 to 40 minutes.

4 servings

Manicotti (Stuffaroni)

Giant tubular pasta shells work well in this dish. If you use manicotti, they can be filled with a pastry bag, or perhaps better, by holding each manicotti upright in one hand, its base resting on your palm. Fill the tube with an iced-tea spoon, shaking the cottage cheese mixture to eliminate air bubbles. The method is a bit messy but effective.

16 ounces plain, nonfat cottage cheese

2 tablespoons grated Asiago or
    Parmesan cheese

2 egg whites

2 tablespoons sauce and gravy flour
    (pulverized flour)

1 tablespoon plus 1 teaspoon fresh
    oregano, chopped, or 1¼ teaspoons
    dried oregano

2 tablespoons fresh basil, chopped, or 2
    teaspoons dried basil

1 tablespoon plus 1 teaspoon fresh
    thyme, chopped, or 1 teaspoon
    dried thyme

pepper

6 cups fat-free pasta sauce

12 stuffaroni

- Purée the cottage cheese, cheese, egg whites, flour, herbs, and pepper until just smooth.
- Put a very thin layer of the pasta sauce into a 9- by 13-inch pan.
- Fill the stuffaroni and place them in the pan in a single layer. Space them so they do not touch the sides of the pan or each other.
- Bring the pasta sauce to a boil and spoon it over the stuffed pasta.
- Cover tightly with foil and bake in a preheated 400°F oven for 55 minutes.

4 servings

Tomatoes and Basil With Pasta

Fresh, juicy Roma tomatoes are essential for this recipe. Best are homegrown tomatoes or fresh Romas from the farmer's market. The simple, untrammeled sauce is best done rapidly so the tomatoes are just softened, not pulpy. This is a midsummer dish, when fruity tomatoes are available.

4 ounces spaghetti or other pasta, uncooked

3 large garlic cloves, minced

1 teaspoon olive oil

1 pound 4 ounces Roma tomatoes, peeled and chopped

1 tablespoon fresh oregano, chopped

salt

pepper

¼ cup fresh basil, chopped

- While the pasta cooks, briefly sauté the garlic in the olive oil using a skillet large enough to hold the pasta and sauce.

- Add the tomatoes and oregano to the pan and simmer rapidly for 8 to 10 minutes, until soft and not wet. Add salt and pepper and stir in the basil.

- Drain the pasta well and add to the sauce.

- Heat briefly and serve.

2 servings

Fresh Tomato Sauce With Roma Tomatoes

Roma tomatoes, when encountered in vast mounds in the produce section, are often uninspiring, hard, red, pear-shaped spears lacking in juice and flavor. Disdain them. Search the farmer's market for some soft, juicy, yielding fruit!

1 pound onion, chopped

1 teaspoon olive oil

5 large garlic cloves, minced

3½ pounds Roma tomatoes, peeled, quartered, and puréed

1 bay leaf

salt

pepper

¼ cup fresh basil, chopped

- Sauté the onion in the olive oil until soft. Add the garlic, briefly stirring.

- Add the puréed tomatoes and bay leaf. Cook for 40 minutes or until thickened. Cover partially to prevent spattering, if necessary, while cooking.

- Add salt and pepper.

- Stir in the basil just before serving.

4 cups

Fresh Tomato Sauce With Romas, Peas, and Basil

Just adding the piquant sweetness of fresh peas to a simple tomato sauce transforms the flavor.

1¼ cups fresh peas

8 ounces onion, chopped

1 teaspoon olive oil

4 large garlic cloves, minced

3 pounds Roma tomatoes, peeled and chopped

2 tablespoons double-concentrated Italian tomato paste (comes in a tube)

salt

pepper

¼ cup fresh basil, chopped

8 ounces linguine or other pasta, cooked

- Cook the peas in boiling water for 30 minutes or until tender.
- Drain the peas and set them aside.
- Sauté the onion in the olive oil until tender. Add the garlic, briefly stirring.
- Add the tomatoes and the tomato paste. Cook, uncovered, until the tomatoes are thick and pulpy (40 to 60 minutes).
- Add salt and pepper.
- Add the cooked peas and continue cooking for 5 minutes.
- Stir in the basil just before serving.
- Serve over freshly cooked pasta.

4 servings

Fresh Roma Tomato Sauce With Sundried Tomatoes

The concentrated tomato-flavor tang of sundried tomatoes intensifies the zing of this sauce.

1 pound onion, chopped

1 teaspoon olive oil

4 large garlic cloves, minced

3½ pounds Roma tomatoes, peeled and chopped

1 16-ounce can tomato paste

10 sundried tomatoes, cut into small pieces with scissors

salt

pepper

4 tablespoons fresh basil, chopped

pasta, cooked

- Sauté the onion in the olive oil until tender. Add the garlic, briefly stirring.
- Add the tomatoes, tomato paste, and sundried tomatoes to the pot.
- Simmer, partially covered, for 40 to 60 minutes or until thickened.
- Purée.
- Reheat and add salt and pepper.
- Stir in the basil just before serving. Serve with cooked pasta.

5 to 6 cups

Tomato-Mushroom Sauce

Choose some really flavorful mushrooms such as porcini, shiitake, or oyster to make this an impressively saucy sauce. In winter, when really good fresh tomatoes are unavailable, using canned provides a very good sauce.

10 ounces mushrooms, sliced thin

4 large garlic cloves, minced

1 teaspoon dried oregano

1 teaspoon dried basil

½ teaspoon dried thyme

salt

pepper

1 28-ounce can crushed tomatoes in purée

½ cup dry, red wine

2 tablespoons double-concentrated Italian tomato paste (comes in a tube)

¼ cup parsley

8 ounces pasta, cooked

parsley, chopped, for garnish

- Sauté the mushrooms in a pan over medium heat until tender and the liquid has evaporated.
- Add the garlic, herbs, salt, and pepper. Cook briefly, stirring.
- Add the tomatoes, wine, tomato paste, and parsley to the pot. Cook, uncovered, for 20 minutes or until thickened.
- Serve over cooked pasta.
- Garnish with parsley.

4 servings

Tomato-Vegetable Sauce

A richly flavored Italian red wine, together with sundried tomatoes and uniformly chopped celery, mushrooms, and carrots, gives this pasta dish a textural and flavor edge.

1 pound onion, chopped

1 teaspoon olive oil

4 garlic cloves, minced

1 14.5-ounce can tomatoes, chopped

1 8-ounce can tomato sauce

1 6-ounce can tomato paste

½ cup dry, red wine

12 ounces mushrooms, chopped in a food processor

2 large celery stalks, chopped in a food processor

1 large carrot, peeled and chopped in a food processor

5 sundried tomatoes, cut in small pieces with scissors

2 tablespoons fresh oregano, chopped

1 tablespoon fresh thyme, chopped

¼ cup chopped parsley

1 bay leaf

¼ teaspoon cayenne

salt

- Sauté the onion in the olive oil until soft. Add the garlic, briefly stirring.
- Add the remaining ingredients, except for the salt, to the pot.
- Simmer, covered, for 1 hour.
- Add salt.
- Serve with cooked pasta.

5 servings

215

Tomato-Wine Sauce

It's the wine that strengthens this dish.

1 pound onion, chopped

1 teaspoon olive oil

4 large garlic cloves, minced

2 8-ounce cans tomatoes

1 2-ounce can tomato paste

1 cup dry, red wine

2 tablespoons fresh oregano, chopped

$^2/_3$ cup fresh basil, chopped

2 tablespoons fresh thyme, chopped

salt

pepper

brown sugar

- Sauté the onion in the olive oil until soft. Add the garlic, briefly stirring.
- Purée the tomatoes and add to the pan along with the tomato paste, red wine, and herbs.
- Simmer, partially covered, for 20 minutes, stirring occasionally.
- Add salt, pepper, and brown sugar.
- Serve over cooked pasta.

6 servings

Condiments

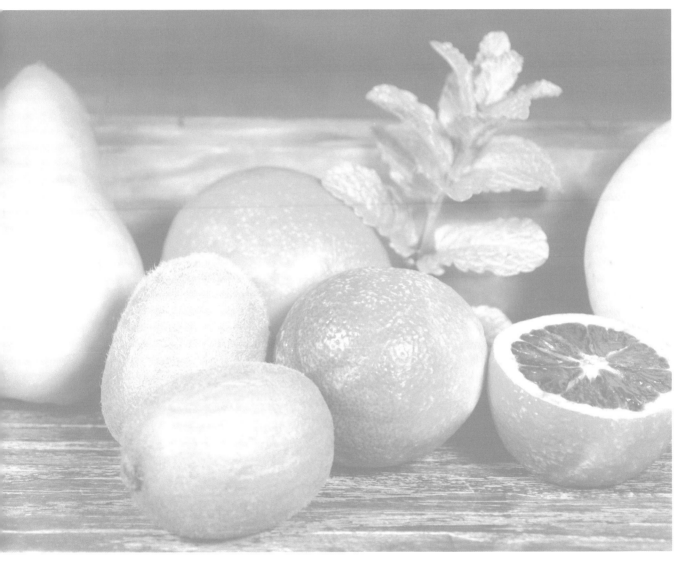

Apples, Sautéed, to Accompany Tofu

Tofu often needs a contrastingly flavored condiment. Chutney will do, but apples, if they be tart, add just the right touch. You might also use organic applesauce.

1½ pounds Fuji or Granny Smith apples, peeled, cored, and cut into small wedges

1 cup or more of organic apple juice

- Combine the apples and apple juice in a large skillet.
- Cook, covered, over low heat for 10 to 30 minutes, often testing the apples for doneness.
- Serve warm with sautéed tofu.

2 servings

Chutney

Why bother to make homemade chutney? Commercial chutney is often too thick and gluey. Further, it does taste like it has lain o'er long on the store shelves.

1 pound Fuji apples, peeled, cored, and chopped

1 pound firm, ripe pears, peeled, cored, and chopped

¾ cup dried apricots, chopped

½ cup golden raisins

3 tablespoons dark brown sugar

1 tablespoon lime juice

2 tablespoons fresh ginger, chopped

2 teaspoons yellow mustard seed

¼ teaspoon cinnamon

¼ teaspoon cardamom

⅛ teaspoon cayenne

1 teaspoon garam masala

¼ cup water

- Combine all the ingredients in a pan
- Bring to a boil, reduce heat, cover, and simmer for 30 minutes or until tender, stirring occasionally.

About 4½ cups

Mango Chutney

This delicious chutney is neither too bland nor too spicy. Use it after one week so the varied flavors can ensemble.

2 mangoes, almost ripe, peeled and cubed

8 ounces onion, chopped

2 teaspoons garlic, minced

1 cup dark brown sugar, packed

½ cup fresh lime juice

1 cup fresh pineapple, cubed

¼ cup malt vinegar

2 tablespoons grapefruit peel, cut into small pieces

1 cup raisins

¼ cup dates, chopped

¼ cup prunes, chopped

¼ teaspoon ground nutmeg

½ teaspoon ground allspice

½ teaspoon ground cloves

1 tablespoon fresh ginger, grated

¼ teaspoon black pepper

⅛ teaspoon cayenne

- Combine mangoes, onion, garlic, sugar, lime juice, pineapple, and vinegar.
- Bring the mixture to a boil and simmer rapidly for about 10 minutes.
- Add the remaining ingredients and simmer for 30 minutes. Cool.
- Transfer the cooked chutney to jars, cover, and refrigerate.

Corn Relish

Adjust the acidity of this relish, if you like, by substituting rice vinegar, which is much less tart, for the white stuff.

4 ears yellow or white corn
6 ounces onion, chopped
½ cup red bell pepper
½ cup green bell pepper
1¼ cups white (distilled) vinegar
¼ cup water
½ cup sugar
¾ teaspoon turmeric
1 teaspoon dry mustard
⅛ teaspoon cayenne
¼ teaspoon salt

- Cut the corn from the ears (2 to 3 cups).
- Combine the corn with the remaining ingredients.
- Bring the mixture to a boil, reduce the heat, and simmer for about 10 to 15 minutes.

Bread and Butter Pickles

Freshly made pickles contrast favorably in taste and crispness with the commercial kind. Look for the pickling-size cukes in a farmer's market.

1½ pounds pickling cucumbers, scrubbed well and sliced ¼-inch thick

1 large onion, halved lengthwise and sliced thin

2 tablespoons coarse salt

ice cubes

1 cup cider vinegar

1 cup sugar

1 tablespoon mustard seed

1 teaspoon celery seed

¼ teaspoon turmeric

¼ teaspoon cayenne

- Combine the cucumbers, onion, and salt in a large bowl and mix well.
- Top the cucumber mixture with a thick layer of ice cubes, cover, and refrigerate for 2 days.
- Drain the cucumber mixture and rinse the cukes with cold water.
- Combine the vinegar, sugar, mustard seed, celery seed, turmeric, and cayenne in a pot large enough to hold the cucumber mixture. Bring to a boil, stirring, to be sure the sugar dissolves.
- Add the cucumber mixture to the pot, stir, and remove from the heat when the mixture just begins to simmer.
- Transfer to a bowl and cool.
- Cover and refrigerate 1 day.

4½ cups

Apple-Tomatillo Salsa

A note about hot dishes: Chilis, or chili peppers (as opposed to bell peppers, which are mild and delightfully sweet and fruity), are hot; that is, they produce a burning, or when diluted or heated for a while, a pleasantly warm sensation in the mouth and stomach. The heat is produced by an alkaloid called capsaicin, which is most concentrated in the seeds and their place of attachment inside the chili pod. An attempt has been made to quantify the heat of these peppers by diluting the hot portions of the fruit to the point of near blandness, producing the Scoville scale. The habañero chilis are somewhere near the top, while Anaheim chilis can be mild.

These fruits, members of the genus *Capsicum,* are New World plants that probably flourished in the wild throughout Mexico and Central and South America. The Spanish Conquistadors must have discovered them and carried them back to Spain and thence to Europe and the Far East. Individual chilis vary in intensity with size, situation on the mother plant, and growing conditions. They are hot, and they like to be grown in a hot climate. My jalapeño peppers, grown in a cool, foggy climate, were disappointingly bland. Try Serrano chilis in these salsa recipes for a bit of variety.

Caution: Wear rubber gloves when handling hot chilis. Do not touch your skin or face with traces of these peppers on your hands.

8 ounces tomatillos, husked, washed, and chopped

1 green bell pepper, seeded and chopped

1 large Granny Smith apple, cored and chopped

4 ounces Maui or red onion, chopped

¼ cup cilantro, chopped

1 jalapeño, seeded and minced

1 tablespoon fresh lime juice

- Pulse all the ingredients in a food processor and let stand for a minimum of 1 hour.

223

4 cups

Pineapple Salsa

What a simple and refreshing taste to add to tofu or tempeh or a tofu burger.

2 cups fresh pineapple, measured after pulsing in a food processor

zest of 1 lemon

½ cup scallions, sliced

1 tablespoon jalapeño pepper, seeded and minced

1 garlic clove, minced

- Combine all the ingredients and refrigerate them for 1 hour.
- If you want an even hotter salsa, add the seeds. Removing the ridges inside the jalapeño will make the pepper less hot.

2 cups

Mango Salsa

Try serving this with tofu.

2 large, almost ripe mangoes

2 ounces red onion, chopped

¼ cup cilantro, chopped

2 tablespoons lime juice

1 teaspoon jalapeño pepper, seeded and minced

- Peel the mangoes and cut them into small pieces. Squeeze the pit onto the pieces.
- Add the remaining ingredients and refrigerate for 3 hours or longer. Remove the pit.

About 3 cups

Tomato Salsa

Jalapeño peppers vary in the intensity of their heat. Removing the seeds moderates the hotness. Removing the ridges or ribs may reduce it further. Some experimenting is necessary to find the right amount of flavor. Jalapeños are not all the same size, obviously. Their origin and probably the temperature of the climate in which they are grown affect their flavor.

1 pound tomatoes, peeled and chopped
¼ cup scallion, sliced
1 garlic clove, minced
1 jalapeño pepper, seeded and minced

- Drain the chopped tomatoes in a sieve, shaking them to coax the juice out.
- Combine the ingredients.

About 2½ cups

Homemade Catsup

Ripe, juicy, preferably homegrown tomatoes make this condiment a stunning improvement over the bottled kind. Try this on a tofu burger.

2 pounds tomatoes, peeled and
    chopped
2 ounces sundried tomatoes, snipped
    into small pieces
8 ounces onion, chopped
5 tablespoons dark brown sugar
½ bay leaf
4 whole cloves
¼ teaspoon allspice berries, ground
⅛ teaspoon ground black pepper
½ teaspoon cinnamon
¼ teaspoon mustard seed
⅛ teaspoon celery seed
¼ cup malt vinegar
¼ teaspoon salt

- Combine all the ingredients in a pan and simmer, partially covered, for about 45 minutes.
- Put the catsup through a food mill and then sieve it, if you want perfectly smooth catsup.
- If necessary, cook longer until thickened.

2 cups

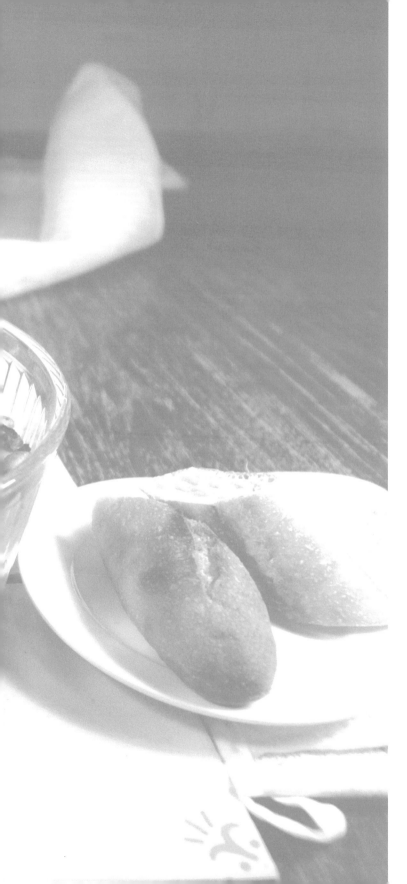

Quick Breads

Low-fat quick breads should be eaten hot from the oven. They are saved from dryness by the addition of fruit: bananas, apricots, apples, even applesauce or berries. Adding nuts, which are now considered nutritionally desirable if eaten in small quantities, adds to the texture and appeal of the bread. Freeze these breads if you must, but heat them in a foil wrap.

The flours for these breads are available at Whole Foods Market stores and through King Arthur Flour (The Baker's Catalogue). Graham flour (named for Sylvester Graham, a pioneering New England nutritionist) is whole-wheat flour that is a bit coarser than usual.

Oatmeal Muffins

These muffins make a marvelous breakfast starter, far better than some of the fake foods and drinks available commercially—the ones filled with high-fructose corn sweetener and huge and unnecessary amounts of synthesized vitamins. Served hot with a steaming cup of freshly brewed coffee, they are a delight.

1 cup unbleached flour
¼ cup brown sugar
3 teaspoons baking powder
½ teaspoon salt
½ teaspoon cinnamon
1 cup quick-cooking oats
⅓ cup mashed banana
¼ cup raisins
2 tablespoons chopped almonds
1 cup nonfat milk
1 egg
2 tablespoons light olive oil
zest of 1 lemon

- Preheat the oven to 400°F and grease 12 muffin cups or use cup liners.
- Combine the flour, sugar, baking powder, salt, cinnamon, oats, banana, raisins, and almonds.
- Whisk together the milk, egg, and olive oil. Add the lemon zest and stir to combine. Add the flour mixture and stir until just combined.
- Divide the mixture evenly among the 12 greased muffin cups.
- Bake for 15 to 18 minutes. Serve warm.

12 muffins

Oat Bran Muffins

Oat bran provides a good source of fiber and protein and can be eaten with soup and salad, even with beans, or for breakfast. These are always best served very hot.

2 cups oat bran

$1/3$ cup brown sugar, packed

2 teaspoons baking powder

$1/2$ teaspoon cinnamon

$1/2$ teaspoon salt

zest of 1 large lemon

$3/4$ cup grated Fuji or other apples

1 cup nonfat milk

2 egg whites

2 tablespoons light olive oil

- Preheat the oven to 425°F and grease or line 12 muffin cups.
- Combine the dry ingredients, lemon zest, and apples.
- Whisk the milk, egg whites, and olive oil together.
- Add the dry ingredients and stir just enough to combine.
- Divide the mixture equally among the 12 muffin cups.
- Bake 15 minutes or until done.

12 muffins

229

Apricot Bran Muffins

Tangy apricots make these muffins. Don't use unsulfured apricots—they look and taste like they should be discarded.

1 cup dried apricots

⅓ cup Grand Marnier liqueur

¾ cup unbleached flour

½ cup whole-wheat flour

¼ cup wheat germ

¼ cup bran, 100 percent natural, unprocessed

2 tablespoons dark brown sugar, packed

¼ teaspoon baking soda

1 teaspoon baking powder

½ teaspoon salt

2 tablespoons light olive oil

1 egg

nonfat milk added to the Grand Marnier drained from the apricots to make 1 cup total liquid

- Preheat the oven to 400°F and grease 12 muffin tins.
- Combine the apricots and the Grand Marnier. Let stand for 60 minutes. Drain well and reserve the liquid.
- Combine the flours, wheat germ, bran, brown sugar, baking soda, baking powder, and salt.
- Whisk together the olive oil, egg, and nonfat milk–Grand Marnier mixture. Add to the flour mixture and stir until just combined. Stir in the apricots.
- Divide the batter among the 12 greased muffin tins.
- Bake at 400°F for 15 minutes.

12 muffins

Blueberry Muffins

Frozen blueberries can be used if fresh ones are unavailable. These are dessert or breakfast muffins and go well with a glass of freshly squeezed orange juice and coffee.

1 cup unbleached flour

1 cup cornmeal

¼ cup sugar

¼ teaspoon baking soda

2½ teaspoons baking powder

1 teaspoon cinnamon

¾ teaspoon salt

1¼ cups nonfat milk

2 tablespoons light olive oil

1 egg

zest of 1 lemon

¾ cup blueberries, washed and
   drained well

- Preheat the oven to 400°F and grease 12 muffin tins.
- Combine the flour, cornmeal, sugar, baking soda, baking powder, cinnamon, and salt.
- Whisk together the milk, olive oil, and egg. Stir in the lemon zest. Combine with the flour mixture and stir until just combined.
- Gently stir in the blueberries.
- Divide the batter among the 12 greased muffin tins.
- Bake at 400°F for 15 minutes until done.

12 muffins

Beer Bread

Try this with a glass of lager and a few niçoise olives or a cup of dark, rich, French roast coffee.

3 cups minus 2 tablespoons
  unbleached flour
4½ teaspoons baking powder
1½ teaspoons salt
¼ cup sugar
1 egg white, beaten slightly
2 teaspoons olive oil
12 ounces beer

- Combine all the ingredients and mix well.
- Place in greased 9- by 5-inch loaf pan.
- Bake at 350°F for 1 hour or until the loaf sounds hollow when tapped on the bottom.

1 loaf

Boston Brown Bread

This bread is delightful when eaten hot with a bit of organic, oil-free peanut butter or jam.

1 cup graham flour
1 cup rye flour
1 cup cornmeal
2¼ teaspoons baking soda
2 teaspoons salt
2 cups buttermilk
¾ cup dark molasses

- Combine the graham flour, rye flour, cornmeal, baking soda, and salt.
- Add the buttermilk and molasses.
- Divide the batter equally between 2 greased 1-pound coffee tins or Boston brown bread tins, if available. Cover with heavy-duty aluminum foil and tie with a string in a bow.
- Place the tins in a large, deep pan on a rack. Add enough boiling water to come halfway up the sides of the tins.
- Cover the pot tightly with a cover or aluminum foil and steam 2 to 2½ hours until the bread tests done. Add more boiling water if necessary.
- Remove the bread from the tins and place in an ungreased pan in a 350°F oven to dry slightly.
- Serve warm or cool.

1 loaf

Rye Soda Bread

Here is a really quick and satisfying bread that gives one the pleasure of handling a pliant dough. Kneading is great therapy, and the bread is rye-flavorful.

2 cups rye flour
2 cups unbleached flour
1 teaspoon baking soda
¾ teaspoon baking powder
2 teaspoons salt
2 teaspoons caraway seeds
2 cups buttermilk

- Sift together the flours, baking soda, baking powder, and salt. Stir in the caraway seeds.
- Add the buttermilk and stir until it forms a dough. Turn the dough onto a lightly floured surface and knead for 2 to 3 minutes, adding as much additional flour as needed to form a smooth dough.
- Shape the dough into 2 6-inch loaves and cut a cross on the top of each.
- Bake on a greased cookie sheet at 375°F for 50 minutes or until done.

1 loaf

Index

Give the Gift of

Vegetarian Revenge

Better Living Without Chemistry

to Your Friends and Colleagues

CHECK YOUR LEADING BOOKSTORE OR ORDER HERE

❏ **YES**, I want _____ copies of *Vegetarian Revenge* at $19.95 each, plus $4.95 shipping per book (Ohio residents please add $1.35 sales tax per book). Canadian orders must be accompanied by a postal money order in U.S. funds. Allow 15 days for delivery.

❏ My check or money order for $_____ is enclosed.

❏ Charge to my: ❏ Visa   ❏ MasterCard   ❏ Discover   ❏ American Express

Name _____

Organization _____

Address _____

City/State/Zip _____

Phone_____ Email _____

Card # _____

Exp. Date_____ Signature _____

Please make your check payable and return to:

BookMasters, Inc.

30 Amberwood Parkway
Ashland, OH 44805

Call your credit card order to (800) 247-6553

Fax (419) 281-6883

order@bookmasters.com   **www.atlasbooks.com**